Empath and Psychic Abilities

The Ultimate Guide for Highly Sensitive People - Includes Guided Meditations to Awaken Third Eye, Develop Intuition, Telepathy, Aura Reading, and Clairvoyance

Nancy Stokes

©Copyright 2021 – Nancy Stokes - All rights reserved

The content contained within this book may not be reproduced, duplicated, or transmitted without direct written permission from the author or the publisher.
Under no circumstances will any blame or legal responsibility be held against the publisher, or author, for any damages, reparation, or monetary loss due to the information contained within this book, either directly or indirectly.

Legal Notice
This book is copyright protected. This book is only for personal use. You cannot amend, distribute, sell, use, quote, or paraphrase any part, or the content within this book, without the consent of the author-publisher.

Disclaimer Notice
Please note the information contained within this document is for educational and entertainment purposes only. All effort has been executed to present accurate, up-to-date, and reliable, complete information. No warranties of any kind are declared or implied. Readers acknowledge that the author is not engaging in the rendering of legal, financial, medical, or professional advice.

Table of Contents

Introduction 5

Chapter 1: Understanding Empaths 9

Chapter 2: How To Discover If You Are An Empath 14

Chapter 3: Capacities of Empaths... 25

Chapter 4: What Is Intuition? 30

Chapter 5: What is Willpower? 40

Chapter 6: Empath Vs. Narcissist... 59

Chapter 7 Self-Development and Self-Empowerment 70

Chapter 8: Mental Toughness 77

Chapter 9: Astral Projection 92

Chapter 10: Psychic Powers and Development............................... 100

Chapter 11: Tools For an Empath's Energy Protection................. 107

Chapter 12 Dealing with an Anxious Empath 113

Chapter 13 Ways To Heal Empaths 119

Chapter 14: How To Cope with Stress When You're Highly Sensitive
.... 125

Chapter 15: Telepathy 129

Chapter 16: Clairvoyance.. 140

Chapter 17: Psychic Ability and Spirituality................................... 144

Chapter 18 Reiki Healing.. 149

Chapter 19 Lucid Dreaming 154

Chapter 20: Predicting Aura 160

Chapter 21: Dream Interpretation 166

Chapter 22: The Chakras 172

Chapter 23: Grounding 180

Chapter 24: Connecting with Your Spirit Guides 189

Chapter 25: Psychic Empaths and Society 196

Chapter 26: Psychic Empaths and Spiritual Awakening 200

Chapter 27: Things that Will Stop you From Enlightenment 207

Chapter 28: The Effect of Awakening 212

Chapter 29: Facets of Awakening 221

Chapter 30: Kickstart Your Psychic Journey 226

Chapter 31: Becoming a Fun Empath 233

Conclusion 239

Introduction

It's a strange world out there. Everyone is just trying to get through the day. We go above and beyond to safeguard our future safety.

Despite the fact that the world is already in a bad state, you will surely face more difficulties as an empath.

Are you an empath, or do you merely attract others who have your characteristics? Whether or not you are interested in the subject, studying the history of empaths might help you better comprehend their current role in society.

Empathic abilities are a gift that is frequently seen as a disadvantage. Those that can empathize will be better equipped than the rest of us to comprehend these situations. Individuals that have this sixth sense are able to tap into another's energy and experience all of their emotions, both bodily and emotional, as well as their energetic state.

At the start of your professional career, being an empath may appear to be a disaster. If given the option, you can choose to "bury your head in the sand." According to certain studies, empaths may find it difficult to function on a daily basis due to the "energetic cacophony" they are subjected to. People frequently experience emotional estrangement, uneasiness, and even a sense of being attacked.

Fortunately, despite the fact that only a limited number of empaths are born each year, empaths are not sentenced to life in prison. Whether or not you believe in curses, this is not one of them. Effective communication skills are an underappreciated asset that can help you lead a successful life if you put in the time and effort. The ability to empathize means that you possess the traits required to operate as a healer if you so desire.

If gathering information from sources we don't understand qualifies as psychic ability, then we all have this ability. Individuals who have had more distinct and consistent experiences distinguish themselves from those who have not.

To put it another way, individuals are hesitant to trust something if they haven't thoroughly examined it with all of their senses. Both an increase in information and greater dependence on what we tell ourselves are possible.

A photographer was setting up his equipment when he was involved in a terrible accident that made global headlines. He abandoned his equipment and fled the area in the lack of an answer. When he returned, he understood that what he had done made far more sense than he had previously thought.

In another situation, a woman felt an overwhelming sense of dread that she couldn't pinpoint but was willing to discuss. Instead, she decided to take a chance. She didn't understand she'd saved her own life until much later when she pieced together the indications she was subconsciously passing down by painstakingly assembling the knowledge she was blind to. This could account for their observations, noises, and scents on both occasions, but the essential thing to remember is that they were fully unaware of it during their interactions.

Accepting that you know more than your rational mind can fathom is a critical step in developing psychic talents.

The purpose of writing this book is to examine how witches' and magicians' psychic powers have evolved over time. In general, this book will teach you how to describe your thoughts, feelings, and ideas effectively and poetically in a range of settings. No matter how much knowledge you have, telepathy will knock you entirely off your game.

Natural skills should be as simple and enjoyable as strolling through a nice, warm, and calm park on a beautiful summer day. Your powers will remain with you for as long as you keep your simple but effective mental barriers in place. People typically rush into developing psychic and paranormal powers without fully understanding the consequences of their actions. You should educate yourself on the most efficient psychic protection measures before embarking on a supernatural journey. As a result, you will always be in a safe environment when traveling.

This book will teach you what psychics are, what they do, and how to improve your own psychic talents. Is there a sense of foreboding in the air?

Using your psychic abilities to assist you in your daily life can be really advantageous. And the more adept you are at connecting with others, comprehending their feelings, and recognizing their joy, the happier you will be.

Psychics are noted for their ability to exist autonomously while being deeply connected to nature. Your hair may appear to have been struck by static electricity because it stands on end. You may have had an odd thought about a friend and then received a text from them confirming it. It is the most fundamental form of psychic ability. As you get a better understanding of the difficulties of control and the strategies for enhancing it, your capacity for control will grow stronger.

We've all heard that psychics are superb communicators who always tell their audience what they want to hear, allowing them to believe all they're told without question. As a result, people are less likely to seek confirmation that the psychic is telling the truth. Individuals cannot determine whether or not a psychic is telling the truth to the best of their ability because there is no way to communicate with the dead or see into the future. There is no way to tell if a psychic is telling the truth or lying because they can only be seen by another psychically talented individual.

When you utilize your psychic abilities to heal another person, the energy you emit is an attempt to transfer healing energy to the patient and their body, which is exactly what you want to happen. Their bodies' energies are being balanced and harmonized, and any obstructions are being cleared, which alleviates discomfort. To help someone in need, the approach harnesses a unique type of healing energy. Psychics can see glimpses of the problem during premonitions, which they can use to find a solution. Some psychics offer clairvoyant health advice to their customers, such as how to improve their health, happiness, and spiritual well-being.

Chapter 1:
Understanding Empaths

It's a common misconception that an empath is simply someone with a high capacity for empathy. Empaths, on the other hand, have even higher empathy levels. Empathetic people can understand and feel what others are feeling, as well as see the world through their eyes.

Sensitive people, also called "highly sensitive people (HSP)," have extremely strong physical, mental, and emotional reactions to a wide range of stimuli. The overwhelming sense of empathy that most empaths experience goes beyond the simple physical reactions that most people have to other people's suffering. The ability to detect and absorb positive and negative energy emanating from other people and your environment is referred to as intuitive thinking. Even if the HSP is no longer exposed to excessive stimuli, re-establishing their equilibrium will take time.

While empathizing can be exhausting, it is a beneficial trait. Individuals with Narcissistic Personality Disorder are diametrically opposed to empaths in every way. Individuals with NPDs are characterized by a lack of empathy for others.

Empaths are extremely difficult to prove or disprove, which makes establishing their existence more difficult. Scientific research is being conducted to determine the root cause of the problem, but so far, only indirect evidence has been discovered. You can examine the brains of people who claim to be empaths and people who claim not to be empaths through CT scans, and you can conduct experiments on people who claim to be empaths to learn more about them. Individuals who identify as empathic but have no idea what that means or who are simply faking their ability to empathize make these studies more difficult to conduct.

We all have mirror neurons in our brains, whether we realize it or not. Compassion allows us to empathize with other people, non-human life, and to appreciate our surroundings. Mirror neurons allow us to gain a better understanding of others' emotional states by using our own as a guide. Empathic mirror neurons are more sensitive to pain than normal mirror neurons. Empaths' hypersensitivity allows them to perceive and absorb the emotions of others and the energies of their surroundings and those around them.

In her research on psychopaths, Dr. Abigail Marsh discovered that empaths are the polar opposite of psychopaths. Marsh conducted a study in which he compared the brains of psychopaths to those of a control group. She discovered that showing the same photographs of people with fearful expressions to both groups had a significant impact on their responses. When it came to recognizing fear and responding to it, the control group outperformed the psychopathic group.

Dr. Marsh chose a group of people who had anonymously donated kidneys. They're known as "anti-psychopaths," according to her research. Despite the fact that she does not use the term "empath," she describes empaths in consistent ways with what we know about empaths. When compared to the control group, anti-psychopaths showed superior face recognition abilities and a greater sensitivity to fear-related facial expressions, according to the findings of this study. The amygdala of anti-psychopaths was found to be 8% larger than those of the control group.

Marsh's research shows the opposite, but it doesn't prove that anti-psychopaths have a higher capacity for emotional recognition and a higher emotional response to other people's emotions than psychopaths.

When anti-psychopaths and psychopaths are compared, the disparity in outcomes is even more pronounced. Psychopaths and anti-psychopaths have significantly different brains than non-psychopaths.

In their natural state, electromagnetic fields can be found in the heart and brain. Empaths are able to act on the information they receive because they have a better ability than the average person to tune into electromagnetic fields. Even when they are separated by a significant distance, empaths are known to be able to sense another person's emotions. It is possible to access the electromagnetic field even if it is thousands of miles away when a person's feelings reach a certain intensity.

They also have the ability to control emotions. According to the findings of the study, empathic people may have a different dopamine experience than the average person. Empaths appear to be more sensitive to the effects of dopamine, a hormone linked to happiness and positive moods, than the general population, according to new research. Furthermore, empaths have a higher sensitivity to dopamine, which has been identified as a trait. They are completely content with happiness equal to that of the average person.

Empaths are people who can sense when someone close to them is in pain or has died before they are told, as well as when something significant or dreadful happens in places where they aren't.

What causes empaths to develop?

They are born with innate abilities. While some people are born with better vision than others, our vision is influenced by our surroundings. From birth, they are hypersensitive to light, sound, and touch. It can be passed down both maternally and paternally.

It all starts with a difficult situation. As a result of this action, they will be more aware of the feelings of those around them, as they will not have the same protective walls as their peers. Parents with Narcissistic Personality Disorder, alcoholism, or drug addiction place a higher value on their children than most parents. They frequently believe that their actions are the result of their own mistakes, leading to low self-esteem. You must prioritize your own well-being over the well-being of others in order to empathize. You have nothing to be embarrassed about. Every child is entitled to special protection. However, it made up for it by inflicting pain on you. Others who are in similar situations to you can benefit from your experience.

Furthermore, positive parenting may aid in the development of empathy, allowing children to become even more compassionate. It's possible that you grew up with a strong attachment to plants. Your parents may have instilled this trait in you when they entrusted you with a section of their yard as a child. Your nurturing and encouragement may have shaped you into a plant empath. It's possible that your natural abilities would have remained dormant if you weren't encouraged early on. You wish to bring joy to those in their immediate vicinity and to serve as a nurturer to others. Empathy increases the likelihood of being harmed by the actions of others. Many empaths claim they are frequently labeled as "overly sensitive."

Many highly sensitive people have an enhanced capacity for perceiving and experiencing emotions (HSPs). Because of their highly developed senses, they may experience sensory overload. They dislike crowds and loud noises.

Empaths are often described as having "big hearts." They frequently bear the burdens or suffer the afflictions of those they help in order to help others.

An empathic person, on the other hand, feels genuine sadness for someone who is bereaved and wishes to assist them. When a person close to them is grieving, they will experience the same emotions as if they were experiencing the same thing.

While not all empaths are introverts, a sizable number of them are. Large groups of people can deplete the emotional energy of empaths, which is why many prefer smaller groups. While introverts aren't always shy or awkward in social situations, it's important to remember their introverted nature. Introverts are often endearing, but they are also sedentary and prefer not to engage in physically active social activities. As a result, extroverts (or people who enjoy being around others) require time alone after an event to unwind and decompress.

Empaths are more likely to notice small details and subtle energies in their surroundings. Even if the sensation is difficult to describe precisely, they trust their gut instinct. Don't be taken in by an empath's warning to be cautious around a specific person.

Empaths are generally apprehensive about being in close quarters with others. Empathy necessitates spending significant time with other people, and when you do, your emotions may be swept up and overwhelmed by theirs. Empaths are afraid of depleting their own resources by assisting others. We'll go over this further in the book because empaths must maintain their sense of self while in a relationship.

People who are drawn to the energy of others and empaths are frequently drawn to each other. Regardless of how much the empath cares about this person, the relationship is harmful to them. When empaths spend time with an energy vampire, their mental, physical, and emotional energy is depleted.

While empathic people may refer to others as "doormats," empathic people would rather suffer than harm others. When confronted with cruel words or actions from others, those who can read emotional cues are less likely to express their outrage. They are not reacting defensively because they are unwilling to take any retaliatory action in response to their treatment. They are not only extremely compassionate, but they can also detect other people's emotions. They are there to protect everyone, so they want to ensure that no one is harmed.

Empaths believe that enjoying and trying to become one with nature is good for their health because it is relaxing, grounding, and energizing.

Empaths are frequently entrusted with the task of providing invaluable advice and companionship to those in need. Empaths are sensitive to other people's emotions as well as their own, which makes them feel better. Friends, family, and professional colleagues may seek advice from people who can empathize and understand the emotions of others. This trait is shared by people who have an innate ability to know what to say or do to help others in difficult situations.

Chapter 2:
How To Discover If You Are An Empath

Determine whether or not you have empathy, which is a necessary component of your true self. Everyone around me perceived me as highly delicate, full of energy, and afraid for the most part of my life (and myself). Things that others found pleasurable or simple, such as scanning large crowds and juggling many jobs, overwhelmed me.

While being meditating in natural environments like forests helped me relax, it didn't prevent me from attracting a lot of vigor and being very active in locations and settings that a "normal" person wouldn't expect.

It was also curious, if not alarming, that if I went out during the day or spent time with someone I knew, I seemed to absorb their feelings. I could sense if any of my buddies were upset about something. Furthermore, if someone was unusually agitated or unruly in the market, I could sense their pain.

If you're reading this, you've most likely been in some of the instances described above and are considering how your heightened empathy could benefit others. Despite the fact that every person's experience is unique, many empaths share tales and empathies.

Empaths appear to have a stronger capacity for empathy than the general population and are very sensitive to both their own feelings and the energy of others. People frequently mix up the phrases compassion and empathy, despite the fact that the two concepts have very different connotations.

Emotional Intelligence Sympathy vs. Compassion

Empathy can be displayed by imagining yourself in the shoes of another person. It helps you to immerse yourself in another person's impassioned reality.

Compassion entails associating particular sensations with specific feelings rather than empathizing with the feelings of others. For example, if a partner becomes ill, you may feel grief or misery for them, independent of their power over you. Consider the following hypothetical scenario: Megan's birthday is almost approaching, and she's invited you and another friend, Claire, to dinner.

Claire inquiries about her willingness to prolong her commitment in response to a request. Megan's cheeks blush as she averts her gaze.

She hesitantly explains that she had to cancel the wedding after learning that her long-term lover was causing her job to suffer.

You immediately feel a hunch in your gut. While Claire offers her sympathy, you try to think of anything to say to console your friend. It appears silly because you are fully aware of the horrible and overwhelming experience Megan and you are currently experiencing.

You excuse yourself for needing to use the restroom in order to keep the tears from falling down your cheeks. Claire appears perplexed by the fact that she is the only one not crying at the table.

Our route through life is marked by innate empathy, which enables us to absorb both positive and bad energy from others. This can be both fun and dangerous.

Compassionate Expressions

Many empathic people make the mistake of believing that everyone else is behaving similarly to them, which is not the case. A number of qualities and symptoms may suggest that a person is extremely sensitive to the energy of others.

For example, the fact that something unexpected does not automatically suggest a lack of sensitivity to the circumstance. The following are possibly the most obvious traits of empathic people:

1. You have a deep affinity with nature or animals.

Animals appreciate empathic people because of their sympathetic nature. Being disgusted by the thought of eating meat is one of the unique traits because they can 'feel' the sensations/vibrations of the food they consume while disgusted.

Outside can assist people in developing the ability to 'energize,' which appeals to persons with sympathetic inclinations. Individuals who are not sensitive label those with a strong connection to nature as "environmentalists."

2. Your levels of anguish, wrath, and loudness are at an all-time low.

Minor injuries, vaccines, and, in general, really unpleasant occurrences might be tough to deal with for someone who is particularly sensitive.

Unhealthy clamors, pungent odors, and even physical contact can all be symptoms of overburdened emotions. An empath finds it difficult to observe and comprehend obscene photographs and videos and avoids internet activity and news reports that represent such behavior.

3. You're still exhausted and nauseous

Many people assume that all medical disorders begin with a painful physiological experience. This is a generally held belief. If this is the case, it explains why many people's empathy remains impeded, as well as why they continue to feel helpless and powerless.

One of the most compelling reasons for all sensitive people to learn how to avoid their negative thoughts having a bad effect on the health of others is the potentially lethal effects that unpleasant sensations can have on one's own health.

4. **People Detox is essential.**

By employing the strategy of detachment, empaths can mitigate the negative consequences of maintaining others' sentiments while remaining linked to them. According to folklore, all empaths are self-observers who need constant solitude from all others. Many extra verses are active and like merging, albeit they avoid it due to the increased size. As a result, people with specific sympathetic traits are more likely to reverse the cooperative link.

5. **Your thoughts are exceptionally active or engaged.**

An empathy test can be used to assess whether a person has ADHD or another impulsivity or centrality-related issue in some instances. When a significant volume of tactile data is introduced, it may be difficult to concentrate on the activities and interests you enjoy and are enthusiastic about.

It's a wonderful place to start if you want to get a sense of how much information your mind has to process on a daily basis. On closer inspection, you'll discover that the vast majority, if not all, of these issues, are either unnecessary or unwanted.

This is a "hardener" state, in which the house (or mind) is overwhelmed with garbage that was not sought. Fortunately, mindfulness and other forms of care can assist you in avoiding this 'drop.'

6. **Your foe is disorganization.**

This is a signal that is not as well-known as the others on the roundabout. To completely appreciate how a calamity flooded with highly sensitive individuals is discovered, one must first analyze the item's essential components.

You almost probably learned about probable vitality at some point in high school or primary school if you took a science class. Even if a component is completely immobile, it has enough life to move.

Empathy can assist absorb the vibrations of objects, just as it can help maintain a person's energy. As a result, keeping your house clean on a regular basis is vital (especially your room).

Not all aspects of empathy can be predicted. Believing that all 'rainbows' and all 'daylights' represent empathy complicates matters for people who really have genuine empathy.

While this may look amazing, empaths are prone to addictions to alcohol, food, work, and medication because these activities serve to distract attention away from negatives and mental illnesses.

There is no justification for this, and the vast majority of people have no understanding of why they binge eat, drink excessively, or engage in other vices. Empaths frequently carry a lot of weight about their centers as a physical kind of 'chocking' themselves against existence's absorbing force.

7. Human Relationships and Empathy

Understanding others may lead us to feel that if we can comprehend them, we will be sensitive and gifted in our jobs as parents and lovers.

Empathy exhibits links that defy their core nature: a flow of life between two people, despite the fact that they quickly become helplessly enmeshed and tied. As a result, it's critical that you only socialize with people who share your enthusiasm.

8. Narcissists and Empaths in a Relationship

Narcissists are looking for empaths. Even when it appears that ardent opposite extremes are constantly attracted, it may be difficult to keep a positive attitude toward genuinely useful individuals and situations.

These folks have frequently commented on vampires' vitality due to their desire to absorb an individual's entire inspiration while avoiding potentially damaging and passionate waste. The narcissistic brotherhood is no different. Empathy seekers who lack the necessary skills to truly protect themselves frequently flock to these organizations. Individuals who were raised in a dependent manner, have a narcissistic parent or have previously been tasked with inflicting pain or grief are more vulnerable to this sort of abuse.

9. <u>Low or excessive self-esteem has an impact on empathy</u>
Empaths appear to be an internal critique for narcissists and other energy vampires who regularly endanger one another. Because of the severe sorrow felt by many people, empathies are especially vulnerable to a lack of trust. Even if the same may be said about tranquility, anxiety, and other psychological issues, most of them can be relieved by becoming more aware of how you see yourself.

Is it Worth It to Take an Empathy Test?

Following the discovery of the aforementioned symptoms, you may come to assume that you have far more empathy than the ordinary person. Empathy, like many other characteristics, can be a sliding scale, with some people being extraordinarily sensitive to the feelings of others and others being entirely uninterested. The empathy test provided here may assist you in learning a lot more about yourself.

Take into consideration the following:

1. Do you feel out of place or as if you don't belong?
2. Do you have an irrational fear?
3. Are you willing to feel another person's or animal's pain?
4. Do these emotions surface in the majority of situations?
5. Do you have an intuitive sense of what other people are thinking and feeling, no matter how hard they try to hide it?
6. Do you (or others) occasionally become unduly excited or sensitive?
7. Do you have ongoing worry or grief that isn't related to a specific situation?
8. Are there any odors that make you feel anxious, such as tears, a lot of development, or specific perfumes?
9. Do you dread open places because they give you a claustrophobic feeling?

10. Have you ever felt completely exhausted after a long meeting?
11. Do you believe that other people's interests influence your personality?
12. Do you spend most of your time indoors composing, writing, or listening to music?
13. Do you keep a safe distance from other people's disputes because they make you feel uncomfortable?
14. Have you ever caught yourself accidentally copying the accents or mannerisms of others?
15. Do you believe it is incredibly difficult for you to do a variety of chores?
16. Do you feel a stronger affinity with nature and wildlife than the ordinary person?
17. Is it possible that individuals may come to you in the future for assistance with their problems?
18. Is it legal to claim that obscene images or recordings have honestly or really inspired you?
19. Do you have any bad habits, such as binge eating, binge drinking, or smoking, or do you indulge in any other risky behavior?
20. Have you noticed any changes in your physical or mental health after taking specific medications or drinking caffeine-containing beverages?

If you replied yes to at least eight of these questions, you might be more empathetic than the average person

What is the most effective technique to deal with empathy?

Empathy exists in the face of both opportunities and limitations, as it does in all skills. Some consider it a blessing, while others consider it a curse. Understanding how to become an empathic person needs considerable work and sensitivity. The information provided below will help you determine how to defend yourself from unwanted vitality and balance.

Your Energy Centers' Equivalence

While many individuals argue over how or why certain people are more empathic than others, many people believe that efficient assimilation of other people's negative energy requires chakra activation.

These seven supernatural vitality residences run in a straight line from the base of the spinal cord to the tip of the spine. At any given time, only one chakra should be open. However, don't go into overdrive. By treating overactive chakras, you can avoid the following consequences:

- Grief and acute loneliness, as well as a lack of ambition and mental difficulty (overactive crown chakra).
- Worry symptoms include anxiety, mental anguish, daydreaming, and nightmares (overactive third-eye chakra).
- Unpleasant behaviors include conversing, tattling, and condemning oneself or others (overactive throat chakra).
- You won't have to deal with others' dependency and put up with a lot while also losing your uniqueness and saying yes when you actually mean no (overactive heart chakra).
- Overcoming challenges with control, hair division, stubbornness, and food addiction (overactive sun-powered plexus).
- Exhibit extreme zeal, struggle with addictions, or struggle to preserve friendships and family relationships (overactive sacral chakra).
- Anger, greediness, and the feeling of being trapped (An excessively active root chakra).

Experts in chakra healing say that blocked chakras cannot heal as quickly as unobstructed chakras. You must alter your vitality community to address this problem.

Techniques of Visualization Should Be Employed

In any situation, empaths may use shield perception to keep chakras clear and active. When you begin to feel anxious, take a deep breath and imagine a wonderful shield or air pocket of white light encircling you (with a certain person, place, or scenario). It should reach a few millimeters past your neck on both sides and cover your entire body. Convince yourself that your barrier shields you against poison, excessive energy, and anxiety. It also protects you from vampires, who take your life energy as a result of their passion.

Although it may look ludicrous, science has demonstrated that the brain and body have difficulty discerning between what we see in our brains and what we see in the real world. This is why considering an uncertain meeting with an untrustworthy life partner, a dust-biting acquaintance, or a family member might elicit a pleasant physical response and joyful responses. You are mistaken if you imagined this shield would keep undesirable vibrations out of your body. Your body will do the heavy lifting for you.

Set your own unique energy limits.

Indeed, even in the face of adversity, one may expect to retain all of one's negative energy. To do so, one must break free from the damaging and well-defined limitations of excitement, both at work and at home.

Examine your feelings and the causes behind them. Pay great attention to your inner world and the factors that impact the fluctuation or loss of your vitality. When you get a caress, ask yourself, "Is this individual perceiving, my presence, or the presence of another?" This will assist you in resisting the urge to react to every emotion that triggers your awareness.

The pivotal point Emptying associations refers to the process of removing people from your life that contribute to feelings of excess or fatigue. Because we feel separation is self-centered, this battle necessitates a tremendous amount of empathy. Keeping one's own energy, on the other hand, is more important than being profound or pompous. It might be tough to feel good about yourself when you work or live with people who make you feel concerned about yourself.

Expensive stones, plants, and even concussions that force earbuds to fall out are all methods for discovering your passionate limits. The use of a weighted cover that fills up and functions as a "shield" has helped me preserve my health and lessen my restlessness.

Working out, being outside, eating delicious food, studying, and testing your thinking, and practicing yoga are all great places to start.

Take it into consideration on a regular basis.

Not only empathy but also thought are essential for everybody who wishes to reach their maximum potential. Understanding this advice, on the other hand, is critical for persons living with the agonizing repercussions of being severely afflicted.

- Improved ability to exert control over one's thoughts and paying attention.
- Thinking in the present helps memory and concentration.
- Enhanced resistance to disease and energy.
- Suggestions for mental and physical health.

Many people are discouraged from thinking because they don't understand why, believe they are religious, or simply don't know where to begin.

Begin by paying attention to your breathing and taking slow, deep breaths while checking or refreshing a mantra or whatever else comes to mind. This assists you in connecting with your (higher) internal identity and transcending your knowledge.

Mediavine.

While it may appear counterintuitive at first, devoting just 20 minutes per day to the aims mentioned above will allow the benefits to surface sooner rather than later.

Another piece of empathy advice is to avoid people who are continually draining your energy and impacting you in an intangible way to the best of their ability. In any case, I believe that making a statement emphasizing not only the significance but also the necessity of this is vital.

Consider the following hypothetical scenario: You are extremely sensitive to ocean development, and getting into contact with it causes your skin to tear, your eyes to expand, and your skin to become damaged. Swimming is your favorite marine activity, yet you frequently finish up cleaning up some seaweed and being thrown overboard.

Swimming with protective equipment and only in places with little or no ocean growth puts you at a safe distance. While you should be aware that a hypersensitive reaction is possible, you should equally be aware that it is common.

It's similar to how coworkers interact with shady family members, accomplices, and pals. Because of their harmful impact, we characterize these people as "poisonous."

Chapter 3:
Capacities of Empaths

Individuals who are empathic in comparison to others have been dubbed empathic. Numerous psychological studies are now being conducted to determine the cause of this. Empathic people are extremely sensitive, and it comes almost naturally to them to sense and experience the thoughts and emotions of others in interpersonal situations. Empathy possesses unique and highly developed features that are valuable not only in your personal life but also in managing numerous families, friendships, and romantic relationships, as well as in business and society.

A person's ability to hear.

Anyone who learns to listen with empathy has an unequaled ability. Empathic listening entails not only paying attention to what is said but also getting "into the conversation" and showing real interest in what is being said, all without interrupting or interrupting the conversation. That is why, by going beyond the words, we attempt to perceive the emotional context in which the interlocutor talks.

This is the only way to get the "whole" picture. Obviously, the more motions you make to express your existence, the closer you are to another individual. Consider the following example: Understanding why a spouse or friend is sick isn't enough; advice and remedies must also consider their emotional wellbeing.

Acceptance of Distinctions

Judging someone has only one effect: it emphasizes differences and alienates others. Because empathic people connect with others intellectually, comprehending their perspectives, situations, and feelings, it is impossible to construct a barrier against judgment. Empathizers do not reject or tolerate difference, particularly when it contradicts their own views or sentiments.

Emotional Intelligence Development

Daniel Goleman is a world-famous expert on emotional intelligence, which was a popular topic in the early 1990s. Because he is entirely concerned with the emotional side of things, he distinguishes between emotional intelligence and cognitive intelligence, which is concerned with the ability to learn and solve issues. Emotional intelligence is the ability of a person to deal with negative sentiments or cravings in a relationship, regulate their emotions in general, and keep good control over himself and his emotions.

Empathetic people are able to empathize with others since they must understand and express their own emotions. Furthermore, good emotional intelligence enables empathy to remain unaffected by the poor moods of others, minimizing the likelihood of ever damaging one's own mood.

Recognize that empathy is a trait that many people share.

1. Empathy is a highly sensitive individual.

If you fit into the empathy category, you've almost likely been told that you're overly sensitive or emotional. Unfortunately, these are the two adjectives that best capture the nature of empathy, which is a pity.

Empaths are also friendly, compassionate, and good listeners. You'll notice a sympathetic friend in your group because he's the one you go to in a crisis because you know you can confide in him, and he'll listen. After all, he is attentive to you, he just has ears for you, and he can provide you with excellent counsel. Caution is advised, however, because they are exceedingly fragile, and due to their lack of protective armor, it is possible to hurt them, even unintentionally.

As a result of their regular contact with others, they are frequently physically and emotionally drained, making empathy difficult to maintain. They must recharge their batteries, unplug from the outer world, and take breaks.

2. <u>They are sensitive to other people's feelings and pain.</u>

Because of their great empathic sensitivity, they have a tendency to absorb the feelings of others without even recognizing doing so. Individuals who are unaware that they act as a mirror, reflecting the feelings of others, may have problems in life as a result of being dissatisfied, unhappy, or furious without realizing it. If they are especially sensitive, they may perceive physiological discomfort and feel bad if the other person causes them harm. As a result, they are more prone to infection and have a lower pain threshold.

3. <u>Empathy is a quality of an introverted person.</u>

Empathy is unsettling in a crowd since it only amplifies the sensations and emotions of those around you. Individuals with high sensitivity prefer to interact with others one-on-one or in small groups, preferably one at a time. Even yet, their duration at a company is limited due to their fatigue from human contact. Despite their superior listening abilities, they are unlikely to reveal personal information about themselves because they prefer to keep their feelings and experiences to themselves.

Empaths like to be alone because being among other people depletes their energy. They are frequently referred to as "solitude seekers," implying that they recharge and rebalance while alone, preferably in nature. If they go out with friends, they arrive independently, allowing them the freedom to travel whenever they want without relying on others for transportation.

4. <u>They are the energy vampires' principal "target."</u>

Perhaps you've heard of energy vampires, those who are aware of the energy they consume. Emotional vampires can diminish the passion, rage, or terror associated with empathy, jeopardizing its stability.

Emotional vampires prey on those who are extremely sensitive because they are incapable of protecting themselves or setting boundaries. The narcissist, preoccupied with himself and convinces others that their own behavior is the root of their issues, is one of the most dangerous sorts of people. In some circumstances, the narcissist will even convince the other person that they are unloved.

5. Nature and animals both adore them.

Empaths are capable of unconditional love, which is why they enjoy spending time with animals, whether they are dogs, cats, or other types of pets. Furthermore, they are incapable of surviving the harm caused by susceptible beings.

You find your equilibrium outside, in nature: you feel especially good by the sea or on a lake because the natural element of water rejuvenates you.

Because you understand that everyone, including humans, has a soul and feelings, you have respect for all living things in the natural world.

6. You have the ability to recognize dishonesty.

Empaths do not need to ask questions, listen to voice tones, or examine nonverbal signs to determine whether or not someone is lying. Their sensitivity allows them to comprehend the reasons behind the other person's deception: malice, ignorance, horrible truths, and so on. In addition to intuition, we have the comfort of knowing why individuals lie to one another.

7. Daydreaming and creative thinking

One of the advantages of empathy is that it naturally makes people creative, talented, and inventive in the arts, which may be very valuable. As a result, they produce exceptional writers, artists, painters, singers, and other performers.

Their proclivity for daydreaming implies that they, too, are dreamers.

If they are not exposed to enough stimuli, they grow bored and distracted. They must complete something at home, work, or school; otherwise, it is difficult to keep them anchored.

8. Violence is inexcusably dangerous.

Physiological and emotional empathy are incapable of withstanding violence due to their proclivity to absorb and experience the pain of others. Nothing comes close, not even violent cinema or news broadcasts. As a result, many people have difficulty reading newspapers or watching television.

9. <u>They are devoid of spirits.</u>

Empaths are rarely seen adhering to social norms. Living in solitude and independence liberates the traditional family from shackles or chains, which is preferable to living in a shared space. As truth seekers, they devote a large amount of time to exploring, reading, and documenting new information. You are so obsessed with information that you are trying to fulfill it to the maximum extent feasible.

Chapter 4:
What Is Intuition?

Our bright thoughts allow us to take the best path, make the finest decision, or devise a winning notion! First, let's define intuition and learn how to use it more frequently.

Intuitive intelligence is exemplified by the nose, presence, sixth sense, emotion, inner voice, instinct, and intuitive intelligence. We all use intuition regularly without even realizing it, regardless of the title.

We can use it to understand the meaning of adversity, to anticipate an event, to perceive one's true psychological or physical condition, to quickly comprehend an occurrence, to make the best decision, to be inspired to anticipate a danger... and, most importantly, to guide us toward greater happiness, thanks to his wise advice!

Intuition gives us a sense of completion; it takes us to a place of inner certainty where ambiguity has no place. Then we enter the flow of life, which is defined by its simplicity and fluidity.

It connects us to the information we keep within ourselves, providing us with a new perspective on life and the universe in addition to its practical applications. It immediately sends us to our right hemisphere, where we may use all of our senses to administer access codes relating to our well-being and health. It serves a specific purpose in that it provides us with the necessary responses that allow us to have enjoyable experiences. Even though we aren't continuously aware of it, we intuitively know what is and isn't healthy for us.

When we say, "My intuition tells me..." or "I know..." we are speaking to ourselves. While we all have intuition at times, it is most visible when we ignore it. Unfortunately, when we examine the repercussions of our life choices, we discover that we were not provided with sufficient knowledge. Recognize that intuition is a natural state of mind that shows itself in the form of sights, perceptions, sensations, and language cues to help you identify and trust your intuition more successfully. It is always straightforward and genuine, no matter how it is said.

We can tell that the knowledge is correct because it presses its way into our brains. However, because it is not founded on reasoning, we must have a great deal of faith and guts to follow it. Psychiatrist Carl Gustav Jung, on the other hand, refers to it as "irrational psychic activity" in his books.

Similar to how Mind Maps connects us to our right hemisphere, intuition connects us to our right hemisphere, which is responsible for our ability to synthesize information and offers us access to the domain of emotions, our five senses, and the material stored in our unconscious. By asking ourselves questions, we begin the intuitive learning process.

At some point, all knowledge is decanted into the unconscious, and intuition emerges in a fraction of a second. To be able to recognize and acknowledge one's intuition, one must first be able to sense it. Intuition is intended to provide us with a reaction, illumination, and advice in response to a certain situation or scenario. At different times, three of our sensory pathways may exhibit a range of expressions.

We all have a preferred mode of perception for a variety of reasons, such as recognition, amplification, and, most crucially, constant stimulation.

1. Hearing is the first of the five senses. The little voice in our thoughts is the one that speaks to us. This mode is especially effective in more mundane elements of our existence. As a result, in order to identify intuition for what it is, we must follow its signal in real life to validate or disprove the reaction.
2. Through perceptions or bodily experiences, the kinesthetic channel takes us from a pleasurable to an uncomfortable state of mind. Depending on the situation and individual, symptoms may range from abdominal discomfort or strain to chest expansion or constriction.

3. People who are prone to kinetic intuition have a strong emotional relationship. Their ability to immediately symbiotically integrate into their surroundings reveals their sensitivity to the atmosphere of any given location or space. Similarly, they can detect the state of another human via osmosis. As a result of their increased sensitivity, they have an unequaled sense of touch and fragrance.
4. Finally, visual intuition manifests itself as visible-to-the-mind flashes. The third channel, as a radar receiver, serves to reflect our observation capacity by receiving data. The intuitive visual may see images, symbols, and scenes.

This form of intuition enables us to raise our antennae, which improves our ability to discriminate, communicate with others through sign language, stay alert, and predict events. Because of this, people are able to "see" events before they occur.

It is sometimes possible to plan ahead of time and make changes or fixes before an issue emerges. Intuition can be a powerful friend. It improves decision-making and fosters creativity.

How do you connect with your intuition?

Our emotions, with the exception of our meditation training, are not the most dependable guides when presented with a difficult decision. This is simply because we haven't fully grasped the ebb and flow of life. We strive to ride the waves instead of being pushed by them. However, we may be able to attain the same result with our ideas.

The intuitive part of spirituality

Take a look at the current situation from a spiritual stance. It's not about establishing the reality of intuition but rather about believing our profound conviction that we're cultivating the fundamental meaning of life and our being on this earth. Intuition is the physical embodiment and extension of our soul's existence as perceived via our earthly experiences.

As a result, it assumes the function of the heart's voice. After that, we tend to humanize it by referring to it as our inner guide, which is erroneous. We are now incorporating a spiritual dimension into our lives, imbuing it with traits such as knowledge, compassion, and divine presence, to name a few. As a result, our spirits are imbued with a sacred proportion. The following are the four intuitive parameters:

- It appears to have appeared from nowhere.
- We're positive it's correct, but we're not sure how.
- Because it is so powerful, we feel forced to act.
- Because of listening to it, we have had fantastic experiences.

As previously said, intuition is a great ally in a variety of situations. Strong listening skills, for example, add to the ability to make the right decisions, spark inventiveness, and provide a quick grasp of a complex subject.

Whether we're changing jobs, starting a business, employing a new employee, looking for a new apartment, determining if we'll get along with the person we met... or simply choosing to dress more genuinely, intuition is the most trusted consultant. Excessive information and data analysis, on the other hand, has the perverse effect of decreasing our efficiency, which in turn reduces our decision-making power. Our reasoning side works hard but weighing the advantages and disadvantages of many solutions takes far too long.

Our intuition permits us to find solutions to issues rapidly, which are then proven by facts. In our daily lives, intuition influences our decisions. We should be mindful that it is more likely to appear when we are emotionally distressed. We rely on our intuitive "radar" to pick up on the smallest cues and respond fast when we're concerned that a sale will slip through our fingers or that our partner may tire.

Similarly, our daily activities and interests show our intuitive nature. Our awareness is heightened during this time, and we have an exceptional ability to predict events with astounding accuracy. Empathic therapists and physicians, for example, rely on their intuition to make more accurate diagnoses and assist patients through therapy.

A project manager will also have a better idea of the impending product. Consider how we want to use logic to handle everything (and regularly make mistakes) while spending most of the day depending on our intuition, which already knows what is right and best for us.

The purpose of culinary and developmental intuitive intelligence research is to gain access to a unique resource that exists in both nature and the human mind and has the ability to revolutionize and expand individual cognitive functions. It can also aid in the learning and comprehension of events, people, and relationships that begin with choices and decisions and advance to problem-solving and problem-solving-related activities.

When it comes to the human mind, intuition is a lethal weapon as well as a powerful intellectual and perceptual instrument that is not bound by logic or rationality.

It is derived from the Latin term *tuitus*, which means "to teach" and can be used to denote "self-education" or "self-education and learning." In ancient Greece, intuition was associated with the Noùs, which existed beyond logic and beyond the senses, physical perception, dialectics, and reasoning. In English, the Gestalt movement is credited with coining the term "intuition" to convey the concept of insight, which is literally translated as Insight. In psychology, insight refers to the significance of a specific type of learning that leads to the formation of habits and the discovery of answers without the need for thought. Thus, exceptional scientific ideas occur from insight rather than empirical methods such as Archimedes' legendary Eureka moment or any other solution or surprising discovery that emerges spontaneously "seeing inside" or via listening to the intrinsic and I AM Intelligence.

- To begin, the answer occurs subconsciously, that is, in a way and under conditions unrelated to the problem, rather than through logical reasoning or mental effort to solve the problem.
- Second, the solution emerges from the excitement and restlessness associated with stressful dynamics, preferably

from positive emotional events encountered during Mental Relaxation.
- Third, the solution generates a pleasurable sensation of surprise, interfering with our conscious thought and almost throwing us out of control while also evoking a sense of reassuring certainty, which may serve to reinforce our faith in our own skills and the course of life.

Intuition, like any other basic human faculty, is "plastic," which means it can be educated or enhanced over time when subjected to significant and visible application. Adopting specific exercises, in particular, can result in a considerable qualitative and quantitative improvement in one's ability to observe people and develop intuition.

Techniques for Developing Intuitive Intuition

1. <u>Self-esteem is quite important.</u>

This is a natural capacity that the majority of individuals are aware of having acquired, either intentionally or defensively. External observation is the process of taking a fresh look at oneself, one's surroundings, and one's environment.

It is feasible to practice it multiple times every day, regardless of your method or frequent expectations.

2. <u>Inability to make a decision</u>

This method is more difficult to perfect than the previous one since the desire to "analyze" information, people, and situations is frequently ingrained that it becomes an automatic response. As a result, the capacity to resist making hasty judgments and maintain a "neutral" mindset is critical not only for developing intuitive intelligence but also for any personal growth process.

3. <u>Consistent Meditative Practice</u>

To conclude and explain, this third method, which is performed in a serene and quiet setting, is a result of the two preceding styles and approaches. There are no time or frequency constraints outside of protocols or specialized disciplinary procedures; however, it is vital to maintain a certain level of consistency in practice, which should be done regularly.

Maintaining a "neutral" position while sitting in a "comfortable position" or lying on your back in a quiet and comfortable environment, awake to the fact of remaining unspeakable, and adopting an observer and detached approach is sufficient to maintain a "neutral" position and thus refrain from, for example, an incessant flow of one's own thoughts.

This technique, when joined with other disciplines, can be utilized to develop a more comprehensive meditation practice that can be changed over time and according to personal preferences, which will undoubtedly arise as new insights emerge.

4. <u>Be conscious of timings and rhythms.</u>
Pursuing a life marked by cyclical rhythms and timetables does not mean a desire to be as boring as possible; rather, it offers order and harmony to your daily routine. Much of it comes down to linking daily chores like eating, relaxing, sleeping, or devoting oneself to certain pursuits with a reassuring ritual and various temporal references, all of which will undoubtedly benefit the mind and metabolism in general.

5. <u>Use artificial light instead of natural light wherever possible.</u>
Natural light has a wide range of hues and a large dynamic range, including iris and rainbow colors. Because the sun emits light at a range of wavelengths, the light intensity and color temperature shift throughout the day. Natural light influences the intake of vitamin D, melatonin, and cortisol, hormones that are critical for the regulation of vital and cognitive functions, including the ability to access and develop intuitive resources. This method entails documenting a person's perception of the day-night cycle.

6. <u>Develop a stronger empathy for others.</u>

Anyone can enhance their ability to recognize and understand other people's emotions, to put themselves in their shoes, and to feel what they are feeling by engaging in self-directed practices.

7. <u>Creativity Is Beneficial</u>

To develop the ability to access one's own Intuitive Resources, training in the anatomical and functional brain areas connected with imagination and creative expression is required. This includes drawing, painting, poetry, and music, as well as more mundane activities such as cooking, decorating, and flower planting.

The Evolution of Your Personal Life Intuition

Many people liken intuition to a flashing light bulb or a sensation they can feel at their fingertips. What exactly does Intuition do? You must make a choice.

Intuition actually leads you down your chosen route, pointing you in the direction of what is most consistent with who you are and how you feel along the way.

Intuition is neither feminine nor masculine; rather, it is a tool that we have all utilized to control our own lives since birth. It is typically a bodily experience, although it can also be a random thought, image, or sound. As a result, distinguishing between thoughts and emotions is crucial. If you have a feeling that something is coming from your intuition rather than your head, emotions, or anxieties, you can be confident that it is. Unfortunately, many people struggle to tune into their intuition because their brain chatter is too loud and takes precedence.

As a result, paying attention to your emotions is essential for understanding and developing your intuition. Assume you see a distinction between two possibilities. Your instincts tell you that you've made the appropriate choice. Contrary to popular belief, the sense of contraction demonstrates that this is not the case.

In most cases, intuition comes before action. As a result, acting on your intuition as soon as it arises is critical; else, it would be lost forever.

Many people believe that by using intuition, they will lose their ability to think rationally. Intuition provides guidance and sensation. The intellect, on the other hand, investigates the facts and methods needed to convert intuition into something solid. As a result, intuition and intellect combine to form a formidable force!

We all have intuition. Regrettably, we are unaware of it. We don't hear it enough because we don't believe in ourselves. How can you trust your intuition if your feelings aren't supported by facts or evidence?

- As a result, you should approach your training with an open mind. Which aspects of your job are you free to pick and choose from?
- Do you have a preference between two consumers who, based on intuition, you believe are your ideal clients?

Simple activities should be done every day, and at least five minutes should be set out for meditation. As the most crucial stage in developing your intuition, reduce your thinking volume and learn to listen to your feelings.

Sensational intuition is a sort of intuition that arises when you are fully immersed in the current moment. It, like a muscle, can be strengthened and made more tenacious by regular training. Train your intention to strengthen it and receive responses to your queries, bringing you closer to the sixth-class sensory individual level. To improve your intuition, complete the following task right away:

- Locate a peaceful spot to sit and place your feet on the ground.
- Inhale deeply and expel violently, as though you were about to extinguish the flame.
- The pattern's repetition will capture your curiosity.
- Allow your energy to flow freely until you feel comfortable and at ease.

You may begin asking yourself the questions you desire and wait for the answers from your intuition.

It not only 'controls' your intuition, but it also assists you in understanding what your body is attempting to tell you as you ask certain questions during this exercise. Because, as we all know, intuition is dependent on our ability to focus. If you want to develop your intuition, you must also learn to pay attention, wake up, and improve your listening abilities.

When dealing with magnetism, use your intuition.

A lot of good things can happen in your life if you develop your perceptive skill. Better decision-making skills enable you to work toward your life goals in a more realistic and timely manner.

You may boost your magnetic attraction as well. If you like, you can visualize yourself as a massive magnet. The ability to attract positive people, events, and opportunities unexpectedly by functioning as a magnet. You must work on yourself and invest the necessary time and effort to do this, as it cannot be done overnight. You now understand what intuition is and how to cultivate it. What are your long-term objectives?

Chapter 5:
What is Willpower?

We are all capable of exerting willpower. Some of us, if not all of us, meticulously examine everything we do and even create a timeline with action plans to go along with it. This procedure comprises a list of everything we'll need, as well as the names of the people we'll be working with and anything else that will aid us in our goal-achieving efforts. Finally, once everything is completed, we can be confident that everything will work as expected.

Then there's the day of implementation. You have an appointment with a customer at 8:00 a.m. on your calendar, but you wake up at 8:00 a.m. You're confronted with a slew of impediments, and before you know it, you've failed to complete even one of the tasks on your to-do list. Regrettably, you are unable to adhere to your schedule. You lose motivation and decide to put off your aspirations. You haven't even considered it after ten years.

What do you believe is the root of the problem? Unfortunately, you are out of luck due to a lack of willpower.

Consider the following scenario: you are a 250-pound man on a diet. So, you start planning your strategy. You join a gym, purchase new sneakers, a workout bag, a water tumbler, and a Fitbit, among other costly products you believe are required to assist you in losing weight. You've summoned the strength to head to the gym.

You go to the fitness center and sign up for your first bike instruction. Your riding instructor, on the other hand, is courteous and does not ask you to match his pace. He believes in your ability to keep the situation under control. You're making progress now, "slowly but steadily."

Three months later, you're still going to the gym. Your riding instructor appeared to be about to give up. Worse, after your workout, you may become really hungry, prompting you to order from a nearby fast-food restaurant and have a 1000-calorie meal all at once.

In other words, three months after starting the gym, you haven't shed a pound. Why? The problem is straightforward: your willpower is insufficient. You are fully aware that you need to lose weight, and every time you think about it, you are reminded of how badly you want to. But what are your heart and intellect saying about it? Be very truthful to yourself. You must be completely honest with yourself. What exactly do you feel? Are you attempting to lose weight?

Do you consider the behaviors you should avoid in order to attain your goal? Disorganization, difficulty managing stress, poor eating habits, and insufficient sleep, to name a few concerns, are all obstacles to reaching your goals.

Do you consider these potential stumbling blocks when making plans? This is obviously not the case. If you are not pushed to your absolute limit, you are more likely to give up and fail.

Willpower is inextricably linked to brain chemistry. Furthermore, it is influenced by our mental activities. As a result, understanding how willpower works is critical because it enables us to detect when it fails.

Every facet of our daily life is scrutinized, as is their impact on our ability to achieve our goals. This chapter will assist us in developing a better understanding of the behaviors we should keep, improve, and maintain in order to enhance our willpower and, as a result, live a better life. When we face temptations, our willpower is put to the greatest test. If you are successful in resisting, you have raised the bar so that future temptations will not require as much effort as the first.

Putting Off Gratification

The concept of delayed fulfillment holds that we must wait to attain or accomplish something rather than having our desires satisfied immediately. In terms of motivation, delayed satisfaction, according to Baumeister's definition, is equivalent to willpower. As a result, speaking up against temptation slows your fulfillment greatly. This can be noticed when a buyer declines to purchase something at a store or when a dietitian avoids the desire to eat unhealthy foods.

The Willpower Category contains the following objects:

We now understand that willpower is a source of strength that enables us to resist temptation, govern our habits, and achieve success in life. Willpower is classified into four categories. Examples include concepts, emotions, impulses, and the ability to exert control over one's behavior.

Thoughts

This is the first indication of our desire to set our differences aside and focus on the crucial tasks ahead of us. We commonly encounter circumstances in which two or more items compete for our attention at the same time. For example, you may be putting in a lot of effort to complete a task while also dealing with a family issue.

Your concerns about your family's financial situation will divert your attention and make it harder for you to focus fully on your task. Because both of these issues are so important, they cannot be treated at the same time, and a priority must be set.

It is not always possible to focus one's attention on a particular subject while ignoring all other considerations. It takes a lot of determination, but the benefits are enormous if you put in the time and effort.

Emotions

Our emotional makeup has a significant impact on our ability to perform anything. When we've been depressed for a long time, it's tough, if not impossible, to find inspiration to work on something. When the winter lasts longer than it should, these people find it difficult to leave the house and engage in beneficial activities. When the weather begins to cool, all they want to do is cozy up on the couch with a huge blanket and a cup of hot chocolate.

Emotions sap your willpower; therefore, you must be aware of your emotions and channel them positively in order to be productive. You get emotionally and physically fatigued as a result of putting on a false emotional front to please others or concealing your true feelings. Allow your emotions to run wild and revel in your newfound freedom.

Impulses

Some of you may have discovered that sticking to a new diet or workout plan requires a significant amount of effort and perseverance. The feature of impulse destroys and terminates such resolves and procedures. To stay on track with your diet, you may have to resist temptations such as sweets or junk food. Many people refer to this as a desire, and sometimes gratifying our desires is the only way to avoid acting on our impulses.

Impulses are substantially more difficult to manage than traditional notions because they are ephemeral concepts that spring into our heads on occasion. However, by adopting preventive measures such as removing or decreasing the cause of temptation, you can successfully reduce the type of impulses you feel. Your inability to control your appealing thoughts, on the other hand, continues.

This is when the power to alter the path of events becomes apparent. Consider your need for chips, but your willpower causes you to consider something cramped, forcing you to yearn for carrots instead of chips.

If you're willing to shift your perspective, you might find yourself doing a crossword puzzle instead of snacking on chips. Willpower assists you in analyzing and weighing the repercussions of your desires, impulses, or temptations by allowing you to reason within yourself or by disregarding your desires, impulses, or temptations.

Managing a system's performance

In this area, ideas, emotions, and impulses are all grouped together. You can use the performance control tool to monitor your ability to concentrate on a certain task. It also involves your ability or willingness to complete a task, as well as the length of time you can dedicate to a task without feeling overwhelmed. Performance management is the most effective method of eliminating procrastination. It completes the assignment and evaluates the available resources, including the length of time required to complete the project. It helps to decrease pessimism and anxiety that might occur when there is a lot to do in a short amount of time.

Each sort of willpower contributes significantly to our entire perspective on how we carry out our projects. Because willpower is a resource, each category is derived from the same source and so is inextricably linked. If you spend a lot of time repressing bad feelings and thoughts, it may be difficult to fulfill your hunger or thirst when they strike. What exactly is the key's nature? What exactly is the key's nature? Use your willpower more effectively and finish your trim faster to achieve a better balance between these four regions.

The Hot and Cold Zones of the Mental System

Walter Mischel's experiment is based on his own notion of the hot and cold brain system. As a result of this idea, Walter set out to define the process that causes someone to succumb or fight temptation. The theory center is intrigued by the complexity of what happens in a person's mind emotionally, intellectually, and behaviorally when they purposefully delay gratification.

According to Mischel, the brain has two distinct processing systems: hot and great. The rapid system processes data more quickly than the outstanding system. Each of these systems has its own set of properties and behaviors.

The most active system in the brain is the emotional system. It's direct, brief, and open to both impulses and reflections. Environmental stress is another factor. The good system, also known as the Know-System, is in charge of and accountable for a person's ability to make reasonable and self-controlled decisions. The cooling system is frequently damaged, which is aggravated by environmental stress.

The heated system develops early in life, while the cool system takes a little longer. As a result, when given the option of immediate reward vs. delayed gratification, our brain systems frequently choose to listen to our hot or cool systems. This concept produced the idea of a well-organized and planned internal thought process, which piqued the interest of academics.

Mischel's fundamental point is that we should investigate how these two states of brain processes work rather than simply their existence. In certain situations, this link is what motivates us to be passionate or rational.

Effects of External Factors on Hot and Cold Systems

As children get older, the cool system takes over as the dominant system, and they become more reasonable and cautious in their decision-making.

Stress

Stress can quickly activate the heating system, whereas the cooling system can normally run up to a certain level of stress before collapsing. When this threshold is exceeded, the system becomes dysfunctional. When people are under duress, they make unreasonable and impulsive actions. This explains why, despite the fact that it is unproductive, students can consume alcohol while studying for final exams.

Temptations

Temptations are always present, and we try to keep track of and control our responses to them. According to Dianne M. Tice and Ellen Bratslavsky, individuals should be encouraged to experiment with mood regulation.

The initial step of slip occurs when a person, such as a nutritionist, reaches for junk food or a smoker goes for a cigarette. This is followed by the so-called "snowball effect," in which the person goes on an all-out binge.

You believe you have breached the rules and do not feel obligated to return at this time. Rather, they persevere and are appreciative of the temptation that has been granted to them. Furthermore, research indicates that rejecting what you desire will almost always result in a negative cycle defined by a lack of self-control.

As a result, delayed gratification and temptation are critical in understanding how our minds and the will function. Acceptance of a technique needs a comprehensive understanding of its logic. Some of the tactics mentioned by scientists and psychologists are listed below:

Plans for the future

This is known as the implementation goal, and it is a powerful kind of self-control. It also keeps your willpower strong when the temptation arises after you've developed an answer. If you're having difficulties resisting the impulse to drink an extra bottle of alcohol during a party, for example, you may plan ahead and tell yourself that you'll want club soda instead of alcoholic beverages.

The major goal here is to prepare for a possible future temptation. This strategy will help you avoid making irrational or absurd decisions. This will eventually increase your tendency to use when confronted with temptations.

Management experts used the concept of planning to advocate the use of a to-do list. You may always save time and effort by not having to figure out what to do next when you have a list of duties to complete. Planning is a technique for bridging the gap between one's goals and actions.

Goal setting

To plan properly, you must maintain a reasonable level of discipline. This will motivate you to persevere even if the task is difficult. This is the procedure for the emergence of new customs. Set clear goals, put forth the necessary work, and stay on track to fulfill them in good and bad circumstances. This will help your body's self-control and willpower muscles strengthen. The more you organize your life, the less probable it is that you will have to make decisions all the time.

When you overlook a certain location, your willpower deteriorates, leaving you exposed to temptation. Each aim should have its own timetable. Plan for reversals and delays in your timeline to avoid being disappointed if you succumb to temptation.

Any contact, no matter how expensive, time-consuming, or embarrassing, teaches you something new about yourself. Rather than letting your mistakes define you, make an effort to learn from them.

We only have so much energy and resources, so we must resist the desire to pursue too many goals at once. Simply select a few, to begin with, and they will assist you in teaching your behavior while also reinforcing your willpower and self-control. Building new habits is essential because if a pattern is established, things will require less effort to complete. This gives your reserve the breathing space it requires to deal with potentially life-threatening situations.

How to Survive Temptation

This is an excellent approach to boost your willpower. Tentation can be avoided by using an out-of-sight method that boosts your preparedness to battle cravings and temptations. If you find it difficult to resist drinking, for example, you can use this strategy to avoid attending parties or events where alcohol is the only beverage offered.

If you have problems fighting the impulse to go online whenever you sit down in front of your computer, you can unplug from the Internet and use the offline features. Tension can be avoided simply acknowledging that if you don't see it, it's highly unlikely to exist.

Sitting and staring at your temptation is nearly certain to lead to you succumbing, but diverting your attention is the ideal mental technique since it gives you more chances to flee the temptation and avoid succumbing.

Adults who kept candies or sweets in their drawers were less likely to eat them than adults who kept them on a counter or shelf above their workstations, according to a study similar to the marshmallow experiment. As a result, every time you are confronted with a temptation, your willpower weakens, and you get weaker. If you are unaware of your desire, the blind and blind strategy will be employed, thereby increasing your willpower.

Improve your perseverance.

If you have a strong willpower foundation, you can control your impulses. Willpower is an essential component of self-discipline because it allows you to focus on what you must do rather than what you want to accomplish.

Willpower is something that everyone has to some extent. If your deadline is nearing, you might be willing to assist you. However, when you initially receive the task and begin working on it, you have greater willpower than when the deadline approaches. While some people are able to say "no" and stick to their decision, others lack the requisite character fortitude and succumb to their wants.

In a building, there are two main power sources. Your resolve will grow stronger with time, allowing you to keep on top of these two challenges.

When developing willpower, you must always be determined to complete your task. You might want a system that displays to you how far you've progressed toward each objective, for example. Goal setting and tracking will become a habit rather than a chore if you are consistent. You'll want to remain with the system until the finish since you know what you'll receive if you don't.

Increasing your self-esteem

Motivating others is actually a simple process. It's difficult to inspire yourself because it's so simple to declare ""I'm unmotivated," the narrator continues. Two typical excuses are "I'll do it later" and "I'll think about it tomorrow when I'm more motivated." It's all worth devoting an entire day to." Because you don't want to deceive them, you're more receptive to someone pushing you to stay motivated or study. You want to be able to brag about your accomplishments to your parents, siblings, and other significant people in your life. As a result, you prefer to prioritize your own desires.

Self-motivation is essential for daily life. If your alarm goes off in the morning, for example, you must motivate yourself to get out of bed. It would be advantageous if you had a clear sense of purpose. You're probably unaware of how frequently you need to motivate yourself during the day.

You may keep yourself motivated by doing the following:

1. Maintain a good attitude. Make a mental shift toward positivity. Others can readily excite and inspire you due to their vigor and brightness. When straining to appear passionate and excited about a task, people may feel silly and stupid. It is, nonetheless, vital to assist oneself in motivating oneself. If you are excited and optimistic about a task, you will be more motivated to put out more effort.
2. Surround yourself with people that constantly put you under pressure to perform. Inform those in your immediate vicinity, such as friends and family members, of your aspirations. Inquire whether they will be able to help you with the project. Inform them that they may need to impose pressure on you in order for you to complete the project or maintain a steady rate of development.
3. Reward yourself on a consistent basis. Reward yourself after you complete a step or a task. After you receive the reward, it is intended to urge you to continue working on your next activity or to make progress toward a new objective.
4. Begin as soon as you feel inclined. Look for sources of inspiration as soon as you begin a project. If you enjoy seeing a project through to completion, starting a project and chasing down your inspiration may be beneficial. You'll

almost certainly discover it since, having begun the process, you'll want to ensure that it's completed.

5. Allow music to motivate you. You may be more motivated to complete your chores if you prefer to work with background noise, such as music. It's vital to figure out whether or not music can help you stay motivated, as well as what kind of music can. Amirah, for example, can focus better on her homework if she listens to music she appreciates. Roger, on the other hand, is easily distracted from his work by music, which he would rather listen to than work. As a result, Roger prefers to listen to gently performed classical or relaxing music.

6. Make a comparison of your performance to that of others. You, like the vast majority of individuals, enjoy comparing yourself to others. You notice your coworkers putting in a lot of effort into their tasks and wonder why you don't do the same. You compare yourself to your peers who have more money, larger houses, and nicer cars than you. You're baffled as to why you can't reach your goal and why you're not putting in as much effort. It is now time to assess your own performance. Keep track of your progress and reflect on who you were before you began your profession.

Keep track of your progress.

It is critical to stick to your approach because it will motivate you to track your progress on the job on a regular basis. As a result, Roger is no longer responsible for evening preparations or putting the kids to bed. Amirah's hectic schedule requires her to work at specified times throughout the day. She monitors her progress just before going to bed because she never knows when or if she will return home.

- Begin with a clean slate but set a daily goal for yourself. This method will help you increase your daily walking distance or training time. The idea is to always start from scratch and create a daily objective for yourself. If you have a Fitbit, you can set a daily target for the number of steps you want to take. You could wish to add 30 minutes to your regular exercise plan, for example. You begin with a zero and keep track of how much time you spend each day at the end of the day. This progression is documented in a journal or using a data tracker.

- Keeping a journal to record one's thoughts. Even if you're sleepy or don't feel like writing that night, you must set aside time to track your writing progress. If you have a lot of goals, you can use the diary as a tracking log; however, you must break them out as you go. If you write too many goals on the same page, it may be difficult to track your progress later.
- A Microsoft Word or Excel spreadsheet. Another approach is to create an outstanding tablet or to begin with Microsoft Word to chart your development. You can generate and keep a system-compatible document on your computer up to date. Consider the following hypothetical scenario: You've finished your workday and want to know when the greatest time is to keep track of your progress.

This may result in erroneous thinking and a lack of focus on the work at hand. When you analyze your objectives, you ask yourself questions such as "What do I want to accomplish?" and "

How do I start my day?" By asking yourself these questions, you may imagine the perfect conclusion. This allows you to focus on your activities and develop a better understanding of the aspects to consider while tracking your progress.

1. Make a timetable and use a time management approach to organize your time. Purchase a planner to assist you in staying on track with your goals. Whether you wish to call your pals for motivation or not, you should write this down as a reminder to yourself. After all, having a support system is critical to reaching your goals. If you have a rough estimate of how long it will take you to reach your goals, put them on your calendar. Make a documented strategy if you want to meet the second milestone in 10 days, for example.

2. Make no independent attempts. You'll need to find a partner that is as committed to the objective as you are or someone to act as your accountability partner. This person might inspire you to keep going and assist you in understanding your progress.
3. As your life progresses, you'll want to keep track of your joys and sorrows.
4. You will be completely exhausted.

You don't want your boss to discover that you're fatigued from a recent project. You must, however, learn to grow as an individual, even if it is in modest steps. Otherwise, you may have overwhelming emotions. You will have bouts of low self-confidence as your thoughts focus on how your goal and failure are not developing as expected.

Emotions and mental activity exhaust us, and it is our desire to finish mental and emotional labor that drives us. You don't have to put in a lot of effort to feel fatigued at work at the end of the day. Employees in cognitively demanding occupations may experience the same level of tiredness as those in physically demanding occupations. It's not a race, and you should never think you're not putting in the same amount of work as someone else.

Another method for developing self-discipline is to work on improving one's own performance. This will need a lot more concentration and work than you are used to. Even if measuring your progress takes only five to ten minutes per day, it's possible that you'll feel overwhelmed when you reflect on your day at night.

You should be aware of the effort and self-discipline required, and the entire process is difficult, but you should not be discouraged by it. Instead, if it works, it should inspire you to put in even more time and effort to improve your discipline.

Regardless of how weary you are at the end of the day, you've made progress and strengthened your self-discipline. Tracking your progress can help you stay focused, which is especially crucial on difficult days when you don't feel like you're making any progress.

If you make a mistake, you can correct it and go on. The secret to loss is to fall as far forward as possible. This means that you are capable of rectifying and learning from your mistakes. Even some of Hollywood's most famous actors were denied the opportunity, particularly early in their careers. Some have no feature films, whereas others aren't scared to make mistakes in their careers. Remember that you are not alone if you fail, for everyone fails at some point in their lives—and it occurs frequently.

Willpower is analogous to physical strength. Regular exercise will help to strengthen it. This fact may be useful in the future. Those of us who believe we lack willpower and self-control should be encouraged by the fact that these traits may be cultivated. We have the ability to bolster and nourish our willpower.

We can also practice self-discipline in specific areas of our lives, and as our capacity improves, we will be able to apply the same self-discipline to all aspects of our lives. As a result, we get complete independence, much like how strong biceps can be employed for jobs other than weightlifting at the gym.

How does your resolve fare in this situation?

Watch a sad movie or video clip that generally makes you cry. Invest in a comedy film that will make you chuckle every time you watch it. Instead of laughing, fight the desire.

If you continue to do these activities, you may find your willpower weakening. Resisting temptations will build your willpower in the near term, helping you to stay sober for an extended amount of time. You can also strengthen your resolve by altering your everyday routine. Your willpower will be temporarily depleted, but it will be regenerated over time and become even stronger than before.

To put it another way, when you reverse the alphabet or count backward by three, you are forcing your brain to deviate from its typical, predictable routine, presenting it with a difficult challenge. Working on your posture throughout the day, avoiding swear words, and attempting to quit smoking have all been proved to boost a person's overall willpower.

Self-control, self-discipline, and willingness

Willingness is the internal impulse that drives you to act, make a decision, and finish any work until it is completed, regardless of internal or external hurdles, problems, or discomfort. It helps you overcome fears, negative attitudes, and laziness so that you can execute additional acts, even if they are tough and painful.

Self-discipline is described as the refusal to accept instant gratification in order to accomplish a larger or greater aim. Rather, the individual can concentrate on the thoughts, attitudes, and actions that will lead to success and progress. Self-control can be demonstrated by physical, mental, emotional, or spiritual discipline. Self-discipline, on the other hand, does not adhere to a restricted or limited way of life. It is also not at all narrow-minded. Willpower and achievement are built on autonomy and self-control.

Self-control and self-discipline are crucial for daily decisions and behaviors. Self-discipline and self-control are essential if one wishes to continue studying, establish a business, reduce weight, maintain long-term relationships, modify a habit, meditate, better oneself, or keep promises.

Increasing one's mental fortitude

Every piece of advice and direction you've gotten so far has been related to using your mental abilities to fight lethargy. Unfortunately, while everyone wishes to be creative and successful, only a small fraction of people are willing to invest in developing a powerful brain that will allow them to control their own destiny.

What is a person's mental fortitude? When faced with temptation or inaction, your mind has the ability to listen to you. It's also a result of your determination and self-control, which you've perfected through practice. In reality, the first two are almost interchangeable, while the third is a synthesis of the previous two. One may easily argue that one of them is insufficient without the other two.

The definition of "willpower."

The ability to overcome immediate pleasure while avoiding temptation is characterized as the ability to attain short-term goals.

Strong willpower can help you overcome bad feelings and thoughts while also allowing you to evaluate them objectively. Many people construct it with the purpose of utilizing it as a guide to help them make decisions and take action.

It allows us to take a breather and reflect, allowing us to consider fresh possibilities. It also protects you from putting yourself in situations that could result in a negative outcome in the future.

According to scientific studies, willpower is found in the right brain, specifically the prefrontal cortex. Will is known to consume glucose, which, as previously indicated, reduces the ego. When this occurs, our reserves are spent, our guards are dropped, and we become extremely aware of our surroundings.

Willpower, in layman's terms, refers to the ability to complete a task despite disliking it. You're probably aware that children who learn to control their emotions as they grow up mature into more stable and secure people with high self-discipline ratings. As a result, academic performance improves, and personal life improves. As a result, the only option for a person to attain long-term success is to exercise self-control.

Willpower is comparable to the brain. When used infrequently, its strength deteriorates. Gradually increase your use to improve your fitness and strength. If you've always lived in a state of surrender, it will be difficult to create strong willpower. Some psychologists compare it to a muscle in that if it is not exercised, it will constrict and shrink.

Without a doubt, self-control is necessary for overcoming anxiety and obsessions, as well as avoiding harmful behavioral tendencies. When you exercise regularly, you get more control over your life, improve your patience and tolerance, strengthen your relationships, and attain better consistency in your efforts. It also helps you control your emotions, reject negativity, and boost your self-confidence and inner strength, as well as prevent excesses and achieve moderation. Self-control contributes to the development of a well-rounded and complete personality.

However, if you want to work, you must put up an effort and be dedicated. Willpower is located in the conscious mind, but temptation is located in the subconscious; as a result, you must constantly work on building your willpower. Here are a few easy ways to gain weight.

At all costs, avoid succumbing to temptation.

Temptation comes in a number of shapes, sizes, intensities, and forms. Everything is a temptation, from a pleasant delicacy to a captivating drama. Make a public pronouncement of triumph over your thoughts and go on to something else. It's likely that you'll fail the first time, or maybe the second, but you'll eventually have the strength to conquer it.

If you fail the first time, try again later.

It has a mysterious quality to it. If it's difficult for you to say no to the cake right away, remind yourself that tomorrow will come. Then repeat the process the next day and the day after that. Continue putting it off until you've determined it's no longer enticing to you.

This is because your mind is unable to comprehend the absence of a reaction. It will agree, though; if you tell it, you will get it later. The temptation has been postponed indefinitely.

Keep in mind that you should not always be denying your own will. The vehemence of the attack is decreased if you constantly deny it the pleasure it needs. It is critical to invest your willpower properly, as it is finite. As a result, we can reach the following conclusion.

Take down any and all tents on your property.

Avoid storing cakes in the refrigerator if you have a weakness for them. Prevent temptations from penetrating your home to ensure that their ploy does not deceive you. If you are concerned, unplug the television or, more precisely, disconnect the cable connection. Nothing is hidden from view, and you are utterly unaware of everything you do not immediately notice (in most cases).

Prepare your body to withstand the consequences of temptations.

You must first prepare your body in order to properly strengthen your willpower. Consume nutrient-dense foods, exercise regularly, and get adequate sleep. Regular exercise can help you better handle stress and enhance your self-control. Simple exercises like walking or rudimentary yoga might help you build resilience.

You can benefit from affirmations.

Assertiveness can help you improve your self-control. If you make happy, confident phrases that you repeat frequently enough, they will permanently imprint themselves on your subconscious mind. The words "I am unable to consume this cheese pizza" and "I am not interested in purchasing that cheese pizza," for example, are not interchangeable. The first represents your limitations, whilst the second represents your confidence. The following statements should be repeated multiple times:

- I am completely in command of my emotions.
- I am completely in command of my activities.
- With each passing day, my capacity to retain self-control improves.
- I am capable of self-control because it is pleasurable.
- I have the ability to choose which ideas and thoughts to investigate.
- I'm aware that my capacity to regulate my emotions gives me inner power.

Self-discipline is an easy talent to acquire.

We refuse to perform a range of tasks in our daily lives because we lack the essential mental fortitude. These seemingly little acts have the power to strengthen our inner muscles and develop us into better persons. We are hesitant to do so for a variety of reasons, including laziness, lack of confidence, low self-esteem, mental weakness, shyness, and difficulties, as well as simple delays. While some of us may have a strong desire to do so, we are cautious and, as a result, miss out on an opportunity we may regret later. Our manner of thinking is crucial when it comes to improving our willpower.

Despite the fact that your sink is clogged with dirty dishes, you continue to surf the web. Don't let procrastination defeat you any longer. Begin with a single spoon and gradually go to cleaning the entire sink. Your laziness has triumphed. Your sedentary lifestyle has triumphed.

A pregnant woman had difficulty finding a seat on the metro. You have the chance to give her your heart, but you are hesitant. Don't. Give her a seat, and you've scored a tiny victory.

You're fully aware that your clothes need to be washed. You are completely correct. Your mind, on the other hand, tells you that you've done enough fixing and that you should relax in front of the television and watch dumb stuff. Put your faith in others rather than yourself. Put your faith in others rather than yourself. You are able to move around and shower on your own. You'll be in such excellent spirits as a result of your regeneration. Above all, you would have defied your own constraints. Consider your surroundings; you'll encounter a lot of circumstances in which you'll have to select between two options: the regular, easy route and an unexpected diversion. Always use a problem-solving strategy. Instead of sleeping in, use the stairs instead of the elevator, and instead of sleeping in, go to the gym first thing in the morning. Each act of this nature helps to fortify your determination. Create a powerful character for yourself rather than one who is at the mercy of your limited willpower. After you've conquered yourself, you can go on to conquer the rest of the world.

Chapter 6:
Empath Vs. Narcissist

Empaths are naturally drawn to self-healing and nurturing, as well as healing and nurturing others. One of the most common is that they believe extensive internal repairs are required.

They are usually tired and exhausted all of the time. This is a critical situation. Individuals are constantly attempting to take an Empath's life by channeling their own energy. Empaths, on average, take on massive tasks and quickly exhaust themselves; rest does not replenish their energy reserves. That is only the tip of the iceberg; everyday life is extremely difficult.

Empaths make excellent listeners and audience members. They are more likely to become aware of the misfortunes of individuals with whom they are unfamiliar as a result of their genuine concern for the well-being of others. Empaths are extremely common and can be found in the vast majority of people with whom they come into contact. When they reach this stage, they begin to instill cynicism in their entire being.

Because they care so much about others, empaths are generally willing to put their own needs aside in order to help others. People are more likely to open up in their presence, and as a result, they are more willing to listen obediently in order to assist someone else.

Empaths need to be alone in order to heal. Empaths prefer to spend their time alone in order to avoid being exposed to other people's feelings and vitality. It's a new beginning for them, an opportunity to try new things, learn new things, and distance themselves from everything that isn't theirs.

Another sign of a sensitive person is irritable behavior. Major emotional outbursts are common in empaths, and they are sometimes mixed in with their normal ramblings and feelings. In addition to being overwhelmed by these disparate energies, they must deal with and make sense of everything that is currently coming their way.

They are especially vulnerable to violence, cruelty, and other calamities. Because the news and newspapers can be overwhelming to empaths, most people with a high level of empathy eventually stop paying attention to them.

Empaths are frequently able to communicate directly with others. Several empaths recently discovered information they were never told about. To predict future outcomes, knowledge, not intuition or foresight, is required, and this knowledge can only be obtained through education and experience.

Regular exposure to open spaces may be overwhelming or excruciating for empaths. Unfortunately, so many people's emotions are exposed, leaving them vulnerable to being picked on by others when they aren't used to it. Empaths will keep a safe distance from this situation, no matter how bad it gets.

Empaths have the ability to "see" genuine and honest emotions, which allows them to "feel" them. If you agonize over something in your life for an extended period of time, people can tell if you are being truthful or not. It's a difficult situation, especially because they're responsible for family and friends.

Capacity to empathize with the physical and emotional anguish of others. Because of their emotional attachment to the sick person, an increase in the number of empaths will result in the spread of a disease that has nothing to do with them. Compassion is best demonstrated in this case.

These are only a few of the many empathic characteristics that exist, but they are among the most noticeable. Empaths can be a blessing or a curse, depending on the measures you take to protect yourself. Empaths can stay safe by avoiding large groups or open areas under any circumstances. In other words, while you can usually avoid these issues, there are times when you simply cannot. Empaths can protect themselves in a number of ways by adhering to a few simple rules. Crystals, meditation, and The White Light of Protection are just a few of the tools I keep in "My Bag of Tricks."

Crystals

Rose Quartz is well known among empaths for its restorative properties, which aid in the development of genuine love and comfort in their lives. This method may be useful for someone who harbors resentment toward something, someone, or even themselves.

Dark Tourmaline or Hematite is also a good gemstone for empaths because it helps them stay grounded in challenging situations.

Other gemstones can assist you in dealing with a wide range of emotions, whether your own or those of others.

It's critical that you guard against having your positive qualities tainted by what you've been taught.

Citrine is a yellow gemstone that can uplift one's spirits. Citrine is useful for treating ailments because it aids in the removal of negative energy from the patient's condition.

Amethyst. I like how it strengthens your instincts, which I believe is essential. With the exception of empaths, the majority of people have enhanced instincts that can help them recognize that the emotions they are experiencing are truly theirs and not those of others.

Finish with a dash of Rainbow Fluorite to complete the look. I believe this is the case when considering an Empath, Rainbow Fluorite, as the mother of all precious stones. This multicolored gem can be used to balance and strengthen your Chakra energy centers, as well as to remind you to keep your focus on the earth.

Meditation

Contemplation has long been promoted as a method of increasing mindfulness in ways that go beyond what people who are constantly thinking are capable of.

Many people are surprised to learn that our bodies are built to naturally adjust in order to maintain optimal mental, physical, and spiritual health. Assume that being out of balance is as natural as receiving the energy of others on a daily basis. It's amazing!

When you are out of balance, your vital energy does not flow as freely as it should. When one is out of step with others, a throbbing, painful ache can be felt throughout one's life. Consider whether you've been out of balance for a long time. As a result, your body will react by causing sickness and illness.

Empaths can maintain their balance, strength, and wholeness by engaging in introspection and spending time thinking about and reflecting on their experiences. Many Empaths, on the other hand, consider it a last-ditch effort if they include it at all to their list of significant characteristics.

A ray of protection that extends in all directions.

If you want to impress me, you should avoid doing things that do not impress you any more than they already do, such as joining large groups of people. Many people employ this technique in various ways, and there is no one-size-fits-all solution.

Before proceeding, remember to take a few moments to rest and relax. Close your eyes for a few moments after taking a few deep breaths. With each inhale, visualize a white light of assurance filling your entire existence, running down your spine and throughout your body. Consider white light consuming your entire body and radiating out throughout the universe. This is the process's conclusion. Close your eyes and sit quietly for a few minutes to allow yourself to be engulfed by the brightness that surrounds you. Now is an excellent time to grin and express gratitude for having just practiced and for being content with your decision to prioritize yourself. Furthermore, you have only recently been entirely protected from all prior negative and unpleasant energies in your life.

Anxiety in the Bodies of Others: The Anxious Empath

The great majority of empaths are anxious individuals. Compassion, according to Buddhist teaching, is the ability to put oneself in the shoes of another and understand their feelings. It doesn't matter if you've ever been through a disaster of this magnitude. Anyone may recognize images of a disaster. Finally, pity is a strong emotion that some people feel more profoundly because of their social relationships (Intense Anxiety and The Highly Sensitive Person). Empaths are those who are influenced by other people's ideas, desires, musings, and energy without even recognizing it. Even if they are capable of understanding and even expressing others' feelings through their bodies, they will never come into contact with this knowledge. As a result, empaths are frequently on the edge of erupting.

Being an anxious empath might be difficult when it comes to revealing one's feelings.

It appears to be a fantastic idea; empaths are nice, perceptive people who make excellent audience members. There is no way to confirm or reject that notion, but the feelings of others are far more important to them than their own. Empaths may struggle to cope with the unexplainable on the planet and, in some circumstances, attempt to handle the majority of the world's difficulties; however, this is not always the case.

Despite what appears to be the greatest benefit of all, empaths must bear the weight of their own emotions just as much as the others in their lives. When people feel motivated to engage, intervene, and dedicate their full attention to something, they know they have been called.

The Empath is aware of his or her own anxiety.

Pseudoscientists claim that empaths have fewer barriers to concern, social anxiety, and mourning than other individuals, putting them at risk. The following is correct, according to psychiatric studies:

- When a person has social fear (SP), they are more emotional and aware of the opinions of others than when they do not.
- Even if you have been directly impacted by societal change, you can still be sensitive to the challenges of others. This is the best conclusion that can be drawn from the evidence gathered during the investigation.
- In socially restless people, a profile of social-intellectual abilities is associated with increased psychological compassion, emotional and mental state attributions.
- If they are emotionally sensitive, empaths are more likely to become ill and suffer the negative impacts of stress, professional burnout, and physical discomfort.)
- People who are self-aware and compassionate may be able to cope with these emotions.

Maintain a sense of self-awareness regarding your emotional limits.

Empaths are born with the ability to heal and are constantly exposed to it, which is why they are called upon to do so. Because this is so crucial when identifying realistic constraints, it is necessary to convey them succinctly and properly. Recognize your limitations and accept that carrying the weight of the world on your shoulders is an acceptable expectation.

Assume you're embarking on a new adventure.

It is critical to keep track of how different people affect your emotions since this information is critical. After you learn how others communicate their sentiments through their body language, you will be able to manage a wide range of emotions that you may experience in a variety of situations with a variety of others.

Find a way to access your power outlet.

Empaths will, for the most part, conceal their own emotions in order to assist others. Feelings frequently establish a method for regularly departing the body. Have a regular workout routine or habit that you enjoy and that will help you feel more confident in your speaking abilities. Under no circumstances should an empty cup be used as a pouring pitcher.

A number of grounding procedures should be used.

When your emotions get uncomfortably intense, take a few moments to focus. Rather than focusing just on one piece, it is more beneficial to analyze and critique a body of work. Keep track of your high points; they will assist you in remaining grounded in the present moment and paying attention to what is going on around you.

Empathy is a gift that those in control of their worries should treasure.

Because of their immense compassion, empaths are usually viewed as a burden by those around them. When you are in unfamiliar surroundings or watching the news, your nerves may be on fire. To make matters worse, you may assume that your grief is causing you to believe that you are the only person capable of resolving the world's problems.

Individuals may experience social discomfort when associating with family members who are also suffering social discomfort, implying a genetic component.

Social stress is caused by both internal and external factors that you may be unaware of. Witnessing someone else's humiliation is likely to have added to your anxiety. Your overprotective guardians may have also contributed to your inability to develop adequate social skills as a child.

- There are also bodily manifestations such as:
- You're frequently perspiring profusely.
- tremors and trembling
- stomachache, nausea, or vomiting
- The heart is pounding.
- unsteadiness or a lack of stability
- an excruciating headache

- helplessness or despair

The most prevalent passionate side effects are as follows:

- When people are in social situations, they may suffer nervousness.
- A great sense of dread and self-consciousness about being examined, as well as apprehension that others will notice your trepidation
- apprehension of being humiliated or degraded
- given considerable consideration to your jitters
- be concerned with drawing attention
- As a result of their anxiety, people are afraid to act or engage in the activity.

Because you have a high empathic sense, you may be affected by the overwhelming and powerful emotions of others in a variety of social circumstances.

When they are terrified or insane, they avoid individuals and situations that make them feel unpleasant. They meet regularly because they stress out too much before meeting, and then they spend far too much of their time objectively examining the clearly awful social situations in which they find themselves and considering whether or not to accept the other person.

Empaths should also make an attempt to separate themselves from the majority of the key emotions that they become associated with when they are in close proximity to particular groups of individuals.

Unfortunately, social anxiety commonly coexists with alcoholism, depression, and other diseases of varying severity. To be happy, you must have stability and wealth. Dealing with the chaos is a critical first step toward accomplishing these goals.

Compassionate awareness enables you to see the world through the eyes of another person while feeling your own emotions as if you were that person. However, each empath has a distinct set of sympathetic abilities that are structured in a distinct manner.

Empaths are classified into six types, as follows:

Someone Who Is Both Lively and Compassionate

The joyful empath is one of the most well-known types of empaths. As a result of these features, it's highly likely that you'll be able to connect with the feelings of individuals around you instantaneously and flawlessly, feeling their agony as if it were your own. To completely transmit another person's emotions, the highly sensitive individual must integrate those sensations into their own emotionally charged body. Consider someone who is sensitive and motivated by emotion but who feels true grief in the face of another person in distress.

Individuals with a high level of empathy must be able to discern their own sentiments from those of others in order to function successfully. You can help others without jeopardizing your own wealth in this way.

Empathic Is a Medical Term That Describes Someone Who Empathizes with Others. Individuals who are naturally sensitive toward others can benefit from the vivacity of those around them. Many persons with this level of compassion pursue careers in restorative health or elective medicine as a result of their compassion. When physical empaths interact with others, they may be able to "feel" their own attentiveness for the first time. It's possible that they'll see impediments in someone's vitality field and understand they need to be remedied.

Others who can connect with people may be able to discern their emotional states, and these sentiments may appear in their own bodies. When we examine the body symptoms that others may exhibit, we assume that having a medical problem is a possibility. Certain persons, such as those suffering from fibromyalgia or immune system illnesses, may find that having a larger field capacity allows them to conserve energy while still having the ability to destroy their own powers when necessary. Furthermore, some planning can help to improve one's ability to repair broken items.

Geomantic compassion refers to a strong attachment to a place or the natural environment. You could be a geomantic empath if you have weird or jittery feelings for no apparent reason.

A geomantic empath is someone who has a strong emotional connection to a certain region. The holiness of a stone, the sacredness of a forest, the sacredness of a place of worship, or the sacredness of a specific zone of hallowed power may all draw you to sanctity. While you may be sensitive to a location's historical background, you may prefer to feel hatred, dread, or excitement in response to events that occurred there. Spot empaths have an empathic view of the world, and they would be disappointed if it were destroyed. They can't bear the thought of trees being cut down or the environment being harmed in any manner.

If you find yourself having this type of empathy, go outside and get some fresh air to replenish your batteries. Donating to a natural cause may also provide health benefits. Scents and houseplants may assist you in relaxing in your own home. Furthermore, rather than choosing more sophisticated materials for your apparel and furniture, you might go for simple, everyday materials such as wood and cloth.

Capable Of Comprehending Emotions Derived from Plants

You are a plant empath if you can sense what plants require on their own. With green thumbs, you may present a genuine one-of-a-kind gift to your friends and family by carefully planting the suitable plant in the appropriate place of your house or nursery. Many empaths pick jobs that allow them to use their empathetic abilities, such as parks, nurseries, and wilderness areas. To begin, if you have chosen a career that involves dealing with plants, you almost certainly have an innate affinity for them. Only a few people can be guided by plants or trees that can be heard and felt directly by the mind.

You'll be intensely aware of how much physical contact with trees and plants you require if you're an empath like this. Profit from the strengthening of this bond by sitting quietly next to a distinctive tree or plant and gradually changing your approach until you are more in tune with its desires and emotions.

The vast majority of empaths are comfortable around non-human animals and are not afraid of them. Even if this isn't true, it's realistic to expect a creature empath to devote their life to advocating for the well-being of our animal companions. Anyone with this ability can know what an animal needs and may even be able to engage with the animal clairvoyantly.

If you're an empath, you'll most likely spend the majority of your time assisting others. To begin creating your blessing, you must first comprehend the fundamental realities of creatures. You should also think about becoming a creature healer and training for it, as you have an outstanding ability to find and treat any creatures in need.

Claircognizant Empaths Are Intuitive and Empathic People.

You will need to spend time with others if you have enhanced intuition and claircognizance abilities in order to learn from them. When you understand what other people are trying to do, you can almost immediately tell if they are fooling you.

Others gain from persons who have this skill since they can wreak havoc on other people's crops and exploit their vitality. When it comes to clairvoyant empaths, their capacity to enter another person's head and read their thoughts is almost usually linked to their psychic skills.

This ability can be utilized to protect your active field from external influences, preventing others from bombarding you with thoughts and experiences.

People who are empathic struggle to empathize with others. This can be perplexing, disorienting, and make you feel incapable of performing even simple activities. Understanding your empath type, on the other hand, is critical in order to maximize your blessings and abilities for the benefit of yourself and those around you.

Chapter 7
Self-Development and Self-Empowerment

Deepak Chopra's revolutionary book The Seven Spiritual Laws of Success offers seven timeless principles for living a life full of affection, fulfillment, wealth, harmony, and delight. Dharma, which is a Sanskrit phrase, means "the goal of our life" or "the motivator of our lives" in English. According to the Dharma Law, each of us contains unique abilities which we can use to benefit people all across the world in some way. Furthermore, the world has a tremendous need for any unusual skill, which must be met by public disclosure of that ability.

We apply the Law of Dharma to our lives by using our talents to assist others and ourselves. When we live in accordance with our dharma, our lives become more serene, graceful, and liberating. This is due to the fact that we are at the very beginning of everything developing in the physical universe - a genesis that is entirely reliant on chance.

Following Your Dharma

Implementing the Dharma Law and ensuring that your life's motivation is met necessitates three components:

1. Recognize and accept your genuine self. 1. In today's cutting-edge world, many people identify with our molded selves' ephemeral components, such as our physique, mindset, accomplishments, and assets. There's a lot more to who we really are than these outward qualities. It is the most fundamental manifestation of consciousness, love, and fulfillment. It is devoid of pollution. Many approaches, such as introspection and yoga, can assist us in developing a greater awareness of our inner selves.

2. Recognize and showcase your distinct features and strengths. When you are entirely focused on demonstrating your ability, time appears to stand still. You become absorbed in what you're doing, and as a result, you achieve a blissful state of unending consciousness. Please keep in mind that your new abilities are in no way comparable to your previous corporate roles and that you can share your one-to-one gift with people from all walks of life. For example, you could be the type of teacher who is eager to connect with kids and teach in a way that energizes and motivates them to learn. This gift can be displayed both in and out of the classroom, as well as with your family, business, or a group of individuals. Make a mental note of the routines that engage and thrill you. Make a list of all the things you couldn't imagine doing if you had unlimited wealth.
3. Make the most of your capacity for service as a human being. "How can I properly exploit my ability for the benefit of others?" As a result, the personality is received by the soul area. You let go of your problems and strife and join the vast field of comprehension.
4. Keep in mind that the law of dharma has the potential to alter over time as you apply it to your own life. When investigating a common assumption, the more clarity and awareness you have, the more probable it is that your aim will become clear. Maintain your sensitivity and awareness, and you'll see an increase in the number of opportunities to fulfill your dharma on a regular basis.

One of the many advantages of living in the modern world is that we have virtually endless options and a variety of resources at our disposal to help us maximize our potential and achieve influence.

Your ability refers to your average competence or traits in a specific sector or action. I understand that ability is composed of three components: gift, love, and ability. You are talented if you have a gift that you respect and continue to learn more about in order to develop your gift. We need to pay more attention to one other's facial expressions.

Your innate abilities are highly respected.

Your gifts are things that were given to you when you were born, things that you can do on a daily basis, and things that are simple for you to do. Some gifts come early in life, while others appear later in life as you age.

Everyone was given a gift when they were born, and our loved ones, children, and people in our community were able to detect our gifts and assist us in dealing with them as they emerged. In any case, there are times when people worry that it will be difficult to find their gifts or that they will have to make a huge financial commitment before they can open their usual gifts.

- If you don't believe you've identified your ordinary gifts yet, consider the following:
- What exactly do you receive?
- Do people truly say things like, "I wish I could do what you do?"
- If you spend a few moments to relax and answer these questions, you might be able to discover what your inherent strengths are.

You can have a gift but not adore it, or you can have a gift but despise using it. It's not enough to figure out what your gifts are; there's another component that can help you bridge the gap between love and other gifts. If you are enthusiastic about what you do and do it really well, you may experience euphoria. Worshiping what you do may also help you stick with the portions of your career that you despise the most. However, I do not want to train people in specific areas, such as material design and testing, but I am willing to tolerate some little discomfort in order to continue with the activity.

Many people work in a career to make a living, but they do not enjoy it. This will almost certainly be detrimental to both you and your supervisor, and you may find yourself dissatisfied or underproductive at your current job, prompting you to leave or change employment after a period of time. Individuals may fall behind in basic physiological functions or participate in an activity that overwhelms them; for example, many people enjoy sports but lack the physicality, physical quality, or donation skills required to compete. As a result, while love does not ensure a successful career, it is a vital component of one.

Consider the following example:

What can I do if money isn't an issue, or you don't have to worry about paying your bills? Allowing yourself to respond to this request may also help you to expand your capacity.

Enhanced abilities

Now that you understand the nature of the gift and compassion being conveyed, we can move on to abilities. Controlling your particular powers can help you become more effective. Learning new abilities can be accomplished through education, mentorship, employment preparation, and self-training.

We practice throughout our lives to improve our skills, and the instruction we receive might come from a variety of sources. Our school gives excellent preparation opportunities, but it is not the only source; our family, friends, coaches, and others in our local surroundings all contribute to our capacity to prepare.

Each action you take at work, along with the encouragement of your manager, may qualify you to attend specialized seminars to advance your professional growth. If you're a student, every preparation or training course you've taken has helped you improve your talents.

My abilities and expertise have influenced every decision I've made. I make it a point to ensure that my managers allow me to focus on developing new talents that will help both the firm and me. If you are unemployed or do not have access to these chances, you can pay for classes or engage a coach to assist you in improving your abilities. If you are unemployed, you can self-train.

My expertise has evolved over the course of my life and now covers, to name a few things, computer programming, video editing, and teaching, as well as blogging and bespoke tailoring. In contrast, self-education provided me with the majority of the knowledge I required outside of school. Self-training involves an understanding of how to complete an activity appropriately.

- Which of your extracurricular activities did you like the most?
- If you went to university or college, what degree or specialization did you study? What was your child's name?
- As an exchange student, what type of exchange did you participate in?

It has a substantial impact on your talents. After that, what careers would you advise young people to pursue as they grow older? Whether you frequently hear your coworkers discussing anything, investing time and energy in someone at their company, or arguing, it will nearly always have an effect on your talents. For example, my father and sister are both fashion designers, which has inspired me to think more creatively. When I overheard my father or sister discussing samples, textures, and quality, I knew how crucial consistency was to my professional success.

If you look attentively, you'll note that the vast majority of them opened, despite their modest size. Others train on their own with the assistance or encouragement of others in their community, while others enroll in elective courses or attend college. In any event, attempt to devote more of your attention to enhancing your overall quality rather than waste time trying to remedy errors over time.

Improve your technological knowledge on a regular basis.

In this section, we'll discuss the significance of innovation in your field of expertise. Every task demands the use of creativity and inventiveness. Consider the difference between your phone today and your phone five years ago; the increase in power and complexity is twisted in both directions. It's tough to slip further behind if you commit to regularly improving your inventive ability.

Making the most of your efforts

Do you recall how it felt to be fully awake and alert? The ability to turn entirely and completely towards who you are, the sense of being entirely and completely yourself. Many of you were prone to such behavior when you were younger. You chased the soccer ball on your bike, went swimming at the lake, or ran with your buddies.

You had a comprehensive awareness of yourself and your characteristics. There was nothing anyone could do to stop him. Accepting full and complete responsibility for oneself. As we gain expertise, it becomes more difficult to recognize and appreciate our innate gifts. It is more difficult to employ these skills and regain control in situations where others embrace us.

Recognize Your Own Strong Forces

The most basic and obvious method to begin fitting your characteristics is to become acquainted with them.

Consider the following scenario: you've spent the last month getting to know yourself anew, or maybe you just want to. For the first seven days of the month, conduct a quality review and completely immerse yourself in the significance of the findings for your life.

The next week, take a disk evaluation to evaluate if your personality qualities have improved in your daily life. Send an email to your friends enquiring about the characteristics you noticed in the third week.

Declare your presence.

If you are aware of your own distinguishing qualities, this is an excellent opportunity to highlight them. It's fantastic to use your skills, abilities, and powers the way they were designed to be used.

Following the cancellation of Walk the Earth, the band published a song that has recently gone popular, promoting their profession. It's a lovely piece of music. The tuning procedure eventually revealed their quality, capability, and zeal.

We must exhibit specific features as a group. If we do not display these characteristics, the people around us and our general surroundings will pass on the mission we have been given on this earth.

What qualities would you like to project to the rest of the world? Take advantage of your advantages. It had all the makings of a nightmare. This is dreadful. In any case, everyone was pleasant to me. This event allowed me to recognize how my seminars and introductions were hidden within me.

Chapter 8:
Mental Toughness

Numerous studies and papers have been published in recent years to investigate what mental toughness is, how it develops, whether it delivers benefits, and whether it is associated with greater performance.

According to a 2017 study published in the journal Psychological Science titled Mental Toughness and Individual Differences in Learning, Education, and Work, Psychological Well-Being, and Personality: A Systematic Survey, persons who possess it separate themselves from those who do not. This study looked at both environmental and genetic influences and discovered that certain persons have a 50% variance in the 'toughness gene.' While the study did not rule out the possibility of a genetic component, it did indicate that "positive psychological characteristics, more efficient coping techniques, and favorable educational and mental health outcomes" were all associated with psychological strength and that these traits could be used to teach "skills" (Lin, Mutz, Clough, and Papageorgiou, 2017).

You are aware that mental toughness is a legitimate personality trait that scientists value highly. Great! But what precisely does this do for you? Much and much.

While various research has been conducted on the phenomenon, a more recent study has focused on how it might be recreated by identifying critical attributes that people who are psychologically tight already possess. Following that, we can begin practicing putting these actions into action. The following are some of the characteristics associated with persons who have shown grit and used it to achieve great things. To be more specific, you can see a number of these characteristics in successful people in your neighborhood. You'll eventually figure out what's going on with them.

You mistrust your ability to achieve. You believe in yourself. Athletes do not believe they have a chance to win, but they are certain they will. A real estate agent does not anticipate them concluding the sale because they are confident in their ability to sign the necessary documents. Authors do not want to miss out on their big break because they believe their work will be published.

Every assumption they make is based on prior knowledge. While thinking like a winner may sound like something, you'd tell your four-year-old, psychologically tough people have what's known as a "winner's mind." They don't believe it's a possibility, desire, or hope, and they don't believe they should "let it be." Instead, they are confident without a shadow of a doubt that whatever they work for and expect to achieve will be realized.

Regardless of what "it" is that you want, it is critical to remove any doubt that something is too tough or that you will be unable to obtain it. Your achievement is threatened when you begin to doubt yourself. Make no mistake: you will not win. Accept that you will win.

You have a laser-like focus.

What are your options if you have a major project due in a few days and need to complete it? How long do you sit, work, and clear your mind of all distractions before you know it's time to take a break? Is it better to open Facebook, watch some depressing videos, and then some upbeat ones to cheer you up until you realize it's lunchtime, then go back, work for about five minutes, get bored, and talk to one of your coworkers? One might easily imagine a situation in which mental toughness is essential.

You understand that the job must be accomplished and continue accordingly. When anything goes wrong, you don't apologize or try to distract yourself. How did they able to accomplish this? How did they able to accomplish this?

They are the perpetrators of the crime. They are the perpetrators of the crime. They realize that deferring will not benefit them, so they don't do it.

You're working to overcome your apprehension.

Professional athletes continue to astound us because they are able to push their bodies to their ultimate limits, which only a small percentage of us will ever be able to do. You understand that the ultimate goal, whether you're jogging down this path or skiing down a mountain, is to reach the belt or the mountain's base. Despite the fact that their muscles are screaming for relief and their lungs are on fire, they refuse to give up.

A connector connects these to the laser's focus component. Mental toughness is described as the ability to focus so intently on a task that you persevere in the face of adversity. Many of us are overly sensitive to pain, despite the fact that it should serve as a warning sign that we are going to injure ourselves. We come to a halt and assess how far we can go before giving up because we feel the end of the world is the least likely indicator of misery or grief. This could result in physical pain during training or mental misery as a result of attempting to acquire a new skill or complete a project. In fact, the data indicates that it may be beneficial to your efforts. By definition, life is erratic. This is a huge reason why it's both delightful and frustrating. This does not, however, imply that you have no control over the issue. On the contrary, because some of what life throws at you is predictable, you may be ready for whatever it throws at you.

People with a strong will make terrific planners. They begin by deciding on a place and means of transportation. Then they weigh all of the challenges and design solutions to overcome them. As a result, people schedule time in their calendars to prepare for unanticipated events. If you prepare for the worst-case scenario, whether you're looking for a job, pursuing a promotion, boosting your child's academic level, or fighting to pay for college, you'll be better prepared when the ideal chance comes along.

This is not to say that people with cognitive problems are stiff or uncompromising. As a result, planning entails being prepared to adjust your course if the wind direction changes. Everything is dependent on an individual's desire to act when and where the action is required.

You consistently make an attempt. Individuals who present a mental challenge are not detained for a week and then released.

Almost everyone has heard about Thomas Edison's famous quip about inventing the functional light bulb. He demonstrated mental fortitude by refusing to yield in the face of adversity. As an alternative, two or three. As an alternative, two or three. On the other hand, twenty. On the other hand, twenty. He admitted that every setback had taught him something useful. Others who are psychologically tough behave similarly. Many of us are terrified of failure because we perceive it as a reflection of our own inadequacies and a location where we must grow.

You are aware that the term "failure" refers to an "ineffective methodology." If something doesn't work, there's a reason for it, and you'll figure it out so you can do better the next time. If you're not learning anything, you're probably not trying anything. You've never made a mistake if you've never tried. Accept your setbacks and use them to propel you forward in order to develop psychological resilience.

They have the guts to do it.

We have limited experience with it because, with the exception of professions dealing with potentially life-threatening situations, it is rarely needed nowadays. To develop emotional resilience, one must first be courageous. But what exactly does this mean?

Fearlessness is not synonymous with bravery or courage; it is the victory over fear. Fear of failure prevents us from doing things like asking someone out on a date, applying for a job for which we are qualified but not qualified, or relocating to a more promising place. Fear motivates us to create fictitious lives.

In today's culture, why can't there be courage alongside fear? Why can't you face your fears, accept them, and go on? That takes guts. Bravery. It is rarely used to rescue people from burning buildings or to bring structures closer to an enemy stronghold. Assume you are an example of bravery, whatever that means to you.

Fear and courage may coexist in your mind. By combining them, you can make one of them more powerful than the other.

Mental Toughness Components and Indicators

Mental toughness is defined as an individual's ability to withstand challenges, pressures, and tensions while still functioning at a high level regardless of the situation. Self-control, devotion, trust, and the ability to persevere in the face of adversity are the four components of mental toughness. The MTQ48 approach measures these four components to determine a person's mental power. This method of assessing capacity is the only one that is consistent, rapid, and precise in identifying an individual's ability to deal with obstacles and pressure in a wide range of settings. The following four aspects, on the other hand, are crucial:

1. Control: Control refers to a person's effect on himself or herself, as well as the extent to which his or her will is displayed. A person who has complete control over his or her environment has the ability to affect the thoughts, behaviors, and attitudes of people with whom he or she shares space. People who are mentally strong grow in stature as a result of their ability to regulate their emotions and use their abilities to attain their goals. They may also have the ability to influence how others react to them, ensuring that they always behave in the best interests of the group.
2. Emotional Control: People who are mentally strong can control their emotions. You can mask your emotional condition from others by putting on a poker face. These people are notorious for being difficult to read and excessively emotional. Their temperament, on the other

hand, is not readily irritated, and they can keep their cool even in high-stress situations. Individuals who are dealing with psychological issues might regain psychological control over their lives. They feel they have the power to influence people and that their actions will have an impact on their life. They believe they are indispensable and have a strong sense of self-worth.

3. Commitment is described as the ability of a person to "stick" to his or her promises and ambitions. People who are mentally unwell are not easily diverted. It's difficult to take your attention off your task. They are entirely focused on their goal and determined to achieve it regardless of the circumstances. They are always present, practicing and practicing, maintaining a healthy lifestyle, and adhering to their routines. They ensure that promises made to themselves and others are honored. You keep your commitments and go above and beyond. When they say something, they mean it. That is the nature of those with strong wills. They are difficult to persuade.

4. Have faith in yourself: Self-confidence is a crucial part of mental toughness. On a cognitive level, untrustworthy people cannot be tough to deal with. To push oneself farther, one must be satisfied with one's own and other people's talents. They do not require permission from others to know what they are capable of because they are confident in their talents. You are confident in your abilities. They are self-assured in their ability to complete and deliver whatever assignment is handed to them. They have firm beliefs and the capacity to put their trust in others.

5. Lack of trust: A lack of trust refers to a person's lack of belief in his or her own abilities and potential. He believes he is the one person capable of accomplishing what no one else can. He believes he has a one-of-a-kind talent in a particular field. He is self-assured in his talents and is constantly pushing for achievement, willing to go above and beyond to attain his

goals. People with mental illnesses gain from this form of personal trust since it helps them to place their trust in friends, coworkers, colleagues, and family members. Individual self-assurance enables a group to work as a unit. They are indifferent to being frightened or deceived by external forces. They have a self-assured manner.

6. Adversity reaction: This component describes how a person reacts to adversity. Is it more necessary for him to overcome obstacles or to capitalize on opportunities? Problems are viewed as chances for people with high mental demands to demonstrate their talents and abilities. Every obstacle provides an opportunity for individuals to demonstrate their abilities to others. People who have a high level of mental toughness are inspired and motivated to work even harder in order to attain their goals. They don't give up easily and are constantly striving to improve. Adversity is viewed as a chance for personal growth and development. They embrace each obstacle with a desire to grow and learn from it, and their acceptance of them demonstrates this attitude. Individuals with a strong resolve can achieve great things. They learn from their mistakes and do not make the same ones again.

Mental stiffness manifests itself in six ways.

Mental toughness is critical in business and athletics since it determines whether a team or corporation succeeds or fails in its endeavors. Mental toughness manifests itself in at least six ways:

1. Accountability is vital in both business and sports. Commitment and connection are necessary in both cases. It is critical to be connected in order to move as part of a group. A player's game, regardless of ability, will be dismissed if he or she does not have a clear purpose in mind. Employers are required to communicate with their employees on a frequent basis. People who have hardened their hearts are more receptive. They reply in a timely and appropriate manner to

their expectations. Leaders must be adaptable to shifting circumstances and demands. If they don't, their company will go bankrupt.

2. Adaptability and flexibility: The ability to adapt to one's surroundings is one of the most significant characteristics of a mentally tough individual. Even when confronted with a stressful scenario, mentally tough people may keep their cool and resist being easily affected. They can provide quick and effective recommendations to address current needs. Individuals suffering from mental diseases should be receptive to new technologies, principles, methodologies, and inventions, as well as fresh ideas. They must be impartial and objective. Mentally challenged people can adapt and make the required modifications if something needs to be addressed.

3. Ethical and daring behavior: Both athletics and business are extremely difficult to master. The competition is stiff, and the climate is challenging. Unethical professional advancement techniques are common among people pursuing advancement in this environment. People who are mentally tough, on the other hand, would never achieve their goals by using unethical tactics. Daring people are those who are psychologically strong. They are unafraid to speak up against injustice in their community or to defend their beliefs.

4. Fortitude: Even when confronted with several challenges and difficulties, psychologically strong people can achieve exceptional results. They are people that are emotionally, physically, and spiritually strong and will not give up easily. To reach their goals, they work harder than anybody else. They are also oblivious to bodily restrictions. When the odds are stacked against them, executives who work hard to keep their businesses functioning are also willing to oppose force. As a leader, you must be firm in your convictions and be fearless in speaking up for what is right.

5. When a leader is unable to overcome an opposing force, his subordinates and position are compromised. Athletes, on the other hand, must be strong both mentally and physically. There is always a lot of training, and if they are not physically fit, they will find it difficult to stay in a game like this for an extended period of time. Even if you are exhausted and unable to continue, you must rely on your strong resolve to 'push' you on; the mind is immensely powerful, and even if the athlete's body cannot, the athlete's mind will.
6. Sportsmanship: Sportsmanship is crucial in both the athletic and commercial spheres. When confronted with a psychological difficulty, a person understands when to accept a loss and when to respect the abilities and understanding of others. Each team member must assist and inspire the others in order to win. And, regardless of the outcome, they will have to either celebrate together or accept defeat as a community. Accusing one another is futile. They also point fingers in one other's faces.
7. Resilience: It is critical to be able to recover from setbacks and adapt to new situations. When faced with defeat, sorrow, poverty, and failure, difficult individuals should be able to bounce back even harder. They must be strong to endure adversity. They should be subjected to a series of harrowing ordeals. You have the impression that something greater awaits you and that, regardless of the outcome, you are deserving of being at the pinnacle of your profession. This type of thought demonstrates tenacity and endurance. Everyone makes mistakes; what matters is how we respond to and apologize for them.

They speak about a finite spectrum of achievement and swear by a set of rules and a way of thinking that should motivate us to achieve equal levels of success.

Simply aligning and reinforcing your beliefs is all that is required for this mode of thinking to help you overcome any difficulties that life may throw your way.

Before we look at ways to enhance your mental health in order to increase your chances of success in life, let's take a look at the lives of some everyday individuals. Including:

1. Your objectives are framed incorrectly. There is a proper way and a wrong approach to achieving your objectives. It is recommended that you use the SMART technique throughout the process to plan, act, and assess your progress. The greater your ability to assess your progress and go into the smallest details, the more probable it is that you will succeed.
2. An inability to manage their time efficiently—Most people fail because they prefer to wallow in comfort and leisure, which causes them to relapse to old behaviors. Time is a valuable resource that cannot be regained once it has been spent, implying that it cannot be reclaimed once it has passed.
3. Considering other people's points of view - if you give people enough thinking, you will most likely adopt their advice. You, on the other hand, are well aware that you were made for a much bigger purpose than your current perceptions. When you just worry about what others think, you lose motivation and become overly reliant on them for guidance, which might lead you astray.
4. Allow unhealthy behaviors to rule your life- Everyone has a dark side, but some individuals allow it to rule their lives. To break undesired behaviors, you must make a constant effort to improve and strengthen your environment.
5. Giving up rather than persevering—To be honest, failure is an awful sensation. Failure, on the other hand, will either inspire you to develop or result in a setback. Many world champions have encountered disappointments during their careers, but they have never let these setbacks define them. As a result, whatever you do, keep going forward in small steps.

The Secret Can Assist You in Developing a Positive Attitude

You've definitely realized that each component of our derailment has a bad impact on our progress. It may be tough to have a cheerful attitude in a highly negative situation. It's much simpler to complain, point fingers, and sink deeper into apathy and despair than it is to act. The fact that so many of us are impacted is very certainly due to a variety of mental health disorders ranging from stress to depression and other conditions.

A writer recently shared a Facebook post with his readers that he had recently read. According to the announcement, around 1,000 new high-wage employments will be created. The jobs are most likely to be in the blogger's nearby vicinity. When his initial excitement wore off, he began sharing information with others who were qualified and interested in the new position. He did, however, return to the Facebook post an hour later and was astounded by what he discovered.

Rather than being grateful for the new prospects, neighbors began to voice unhappiness with the offices' placement. The public was shocked by the amount of government spending required to allow the well-known firm to function in the newly created space. Others questioned the legitimacy of the posts, considering the region's record-high unemployment rate.

Despite the fact that the posts contained exciting information, the majority of readers were only concerned with the project's costs and other negative aspects, rather than being pleased that the new company was assisting in alleviating local unemployment problems, as the blogger had predicted. The blogger was surprised to learn he had behaved just like the folks he had chastised: he had only read the negative comments and disregarded the positive ones praising the development.

This story demonstrates how success can be classified as either good or negative. What you focus your attention on determines whether you succeed or fail. Those who are psychologically robust, who can adapt to the uncomfortable while recognizing the positive, will prosper. In this context, success is defined as the ability to live a life free of negative influences, culminating in long-term happiness.

Mental toughness benefits everyone, not just athletes. This is true in all aspects of life. To reach this goal, you must apply the eight lessons listed below:

When you're attempting to complete a task, time is against you. You just have a few possibilities, and those options aren't infinite. As a result, cognitively challenged individuals will spend their limited time considering rather than responding. Almost sure you will encounter issues during the performance. Respond positively and get back on track as soon as possible if this occurs. Be cheery instead of complaining, moaning, or criticizing.

A mentally tough individual acts as though he has control over his environment, even if he does not.

Control is not a matter of chance; even in times of crisis, a solution is almost always found. A psychologically tough person, on the other hand, will endure in the face of adversity.

If a person wants to be successful, he or she must believe that they will succeed even if they make mistakes or fail. This trust can be established as a result of a strong mind that believes in its own potential to overcome, even when the situation is really difficult.

Individuals who believe in their own abilities contribute significantly to this degree of trust. Negative people, on the other hand, do nothing but lower your self-esteem and reduce your prospects of success.

You, like everyone else, make mistakes. Hardhearted people, on the other hand, do not let their blunders succeed. Worrying about, reviving, and dwelling on mistakes not only accomplishes nothing but also prevents you from detecting them. Choose a happy medium in which you remember just enough about them to grasp the lessons they taught you. Allow your former self to affect you, but don't let it define you.

If you have mental toughness, you can concentrate and avoid distractions. You recognize that significant accomplishments do not occur overnight. If you continue to commit all of your energy and concentration to one task, you will almost certainly comprehend something that others do not. Without putting in numerous hours of effort, bikers and other athletes are unlikely to achieve their current levels of achievement. Regardless, they accepted and triumphed over their circumstances. Successful people aren't always looking for easier ways to accomplish their goals; in fact, they are pleased with where they are right now.

People who are successful are open to a wide range of chances. Many of these paths are less well-traveled, which can be scary. It takes a strong mind to overcome apprehension, navigate known territory, and construct a new path forward. An achiever is not limited by traditional thinking; rather, it seeks out new options that may lead to new ideas and actions.

It's natural to have doubts about your activities while you're in unfamiliar territory, especially if you lack mental fortitude. The vast majority of people who express a desire to reintegrate into society think they have the authority to accomplish it. The desire to give back improves your mental fortitude by motivating you to make constructive efforts. Volunteering, for example, can boost your confidence while simultaneously increasing your sense of connectedness with others, lessening your risk of unhappiness and loneliness. It is also possible to strengthen one's mental power as a result of the generosity of people who help.

Every day, new technological distractions emerge in the form of live conversations with friends, YouTube videos, emails, text messages, and news feeds. As long as you engage with people, you will periodically succumb to these distractions. A strong brain is capable of filtering out background noise and allowing a person to focus on what is truly important. Even if a person is bored, he or she must put down the phone, switch off notifications, and stop themselves from using the gadget for a period of time.

Your mental fortitude will inspire you to return to your desk after recess or to stop a conversation with a buddy so that you may return to your desk and begin the day's work.

As you can see, great achievement needs top performance. With so many distractions, it may be tough to maintain mental focus on the secret.

To be successful in life, you must first improve your mental fortitude. To begin, you must learn how to organize your feelings and emotions effectively. When you label your emotions, they lose their power.

As a result, if you're experiencing negative emotions, determine whether they're the result of worry, fear, despair, or rage. It is also critical to evaluate how a particular emotion affects your professional performance. Is it possible that stress, for example, promotes people to take irrational risks? Do you intend to act on your whims?

When you are aware of your emotions, you are less likely to act unreasonably since you are aware of your motives.

Second, in order to transcend painful feelings, a new, healthy attitude toward them must be developed. Recognizing and expressing your sentiments isn't enough to link them to the abilities required to regulate them. To give an outlet for your emotions, you'll need an efficient coping approach.

To avoid the problem, some people are resorting to dangerous coping mechanisms such as overcrowding in restaurants, drinking, venting, or staying at home. While these solutions may provide temporary respite, the problems will almost certainly recur in the future. Consider those who will benefit you in the long run rather than those who will harm your relationships, health, or ability to complete duties.

To determine which technique is ideal for you, try out a few different approaches until you find one that works for you. Meditation, exercise, alone time in nature, and many forms of art are all examples of such tactics.

Third, make a concerted effort to break free from any negative thinking patterns you've formed. As a result, when you begin to think thoughts like "I'm such a stupid," you lose the ability to shift your mental habit. As a result, in order to cultivate a hard-won mentality, you must constantly examine your thoughts, recognize patterns and subjects, and refrain from speaking negatively.

When you have an illogical or inefficient thought, respond with something productive. As a result, rather than worrying about how embarrassed you will be giving the presentation, consider it an opportunity to demonstrate your public speaking skills or creative abilities by proposing unique solutions to the problem. By repeating the technique, you can train your brain to think in this manner on a regular basis. Finally, complete the most difficult tasks while maintaining consistency in your operations. You'll realize you have far more power than you ever imagined.

Chapter 9:
Astral Projection

We have the potential to project ourselves out of our physical bodies while sleeping, a process known as astral projection. Despite the fact that they appear far-fetched and perhaps even a little realistic, some scientific literature has documented some successful occurrences of real-world astral projection. As you sleep or meditate intensely, your soul (or astral body) disappears and returns to your physical body. After your spirit has been ejected from your body, you are free to roam wherever you desire.

According to Healthline, unlike astral projections, out-of-body experiences (OBEs) are frequently unplanned. To begin, when someone has an out-of-body experience, their spirit or consciousness floats above and around their body. In contrast, with projections, the consciousness is actively guided to a different area. Second, while astral projection is largely a spiritual practice, out-of-body experiences have been primarily recognized in the medical field.

Astral projection is not a new concept. Its roots can be traced back to prehistoric periods on all continents. According to Shamans and New Agers, astral projections for spiritual wellness and self-care have been practiced for thousands of years by people from a wide range of religious and civilizational backgrounds. Although astral projection has been performed for hundreds of years, it requires a high level of concentration and desire to be successful. Individuals who lack this ability may lose control while astral projecting, which can have disastrous results in some situations.

The subject of whether or not astral projection is a safe technique is frequently raised. When it comes to astral projection, the answer is the same as it is for any other dangerous sport: if done with caution, preparation, and information beforehand, it is absolutely safe. In some situations, astral projections, on the other hand, may be harmful. In contrast, astral projection can be completely safe and even useful! Consider whether you'd like to learn something new that you haven't before. Because astral projections affect both your physical body and your soul, you may suffer from severe psychological and physical consequences in this situation.

Consider astral projection to be a sport or something similar in terms of accessibility. Almost everyone can prepare to project astrologically with proper knowledge and caution. Furthermore, when it comes to astral projection, some persons will naturally require less time and effort to achieve the same results as others.

The following recommendations may be useful: You have a lot of patience. While it's reasonable to desire to practice astral projection in real life from time to time, you should always follow your instincts and wait until you've mastered all of the delicate details of astral projection. For people who don't have the patience to be guided repeatedly during the learning process, astral projection may not be the best option right now.

Mastering the technique of astral projection will take a long time. It will take time to learn, practice, and experiment with different methods; you will not do everything right the first time. If you don't give up after one or two false attempts, you'll almost likely learn how to project correctly in the end. To maximize the benefit of your desired study, you must guarantee that you have the time to commit to it.

According to studies, people aged 13 to 18 have a natural advantage when it comes to astral projection. This is not to say that older individuals can't learn to project; rather, it implies that young people are more receptive, making it easier for them to suspend disbelief and learn about astral projections.

Even if you are well-versed in the specifics of what astral projection is and how to perform it, your preliminary efforts may not be successful, no matter how much and how hard you try. That is why you should experiment with various tactics, strategies, and approaches. If your first attempts at achievement fail, keep trying. This attempt was not overlooked. They just served to prepare you for the next level when you will be able to command your spirit beyond the boundaries of your physical body. You can only learn how to perform anything correctly if you practice it. There are no other options for learning. There are various erroneous methods for avoiding astral projections, and practice and experimentation are your best friends.

Simply follow the path that has been laid out for you, and you will be able to accomplish your goals in no time. It's possible that the journey will be challenging and frustrating. If your efforts irritate or overwhelm you, your genuine desire to learn will be the only thing keeping you going. But don't be alarmed. Maintain your momentum, and you will succeed!

It's a good idea to experiment with projection first if you suspect something will be tough before you begin studying it. Despite the fact that they are all true, a number of incidents have been treated with skepticism.

The scenario is essentially similar when it comes to astral projections. If you went into the experiment with preconceived assumptions about why astral projections are false and then sought to justify your intuition, you would fail terribly. You're making an attempt to refute a claim made by tens of thousands of other people. If you approach this with an open mind and allow yourself to investigate and experiment with new ideas, you will greatly increase your chances of success.

The Methodology of Astral Screening

Not only must you prepare yourself and your thoughts for astral projections, but you must also create a receptive environment. Here are a few basic techniques to make a projection-friendly environment:

Choose a location.

To begin, think about the fundamentals: where do you anticipate often locating your projects? In terms of transportation, how accessible is it?

Your bed: You may discover that projecting from your bed is the most convenient alternative. This atmosphere will not tense your muscles, and it is one in which you are already comfortable and secure in your ability to operate. Furthermore, many individuals prefer to finish watching movies right before going to bed, which is why beds are a better option than sofas. Furthermore, unlike in other more limited situations where you can project, if you are lying in bed, you are not concerned about your body falling out. However, there are certain disadvantages to sleeping on your bed that should be considered in addition to the benefits. In this case, you may be able to put your body to sleep before it separates from your soul if you do it from your bed, as this is the location your body naturally associates with sleeping. Furthermore, if you share a bed with another person, it may not be the best place to sleep because the other person may interfere with your projection efforts on purpose or inadvertently.

If you choose this place, your living room sofa will be an outstanding choice for your specified space, mostly since you will be able to layout it for your convenience. This means that your body may develop a psychological attachment to the area to the point where it feels as though it is sitting on its sofa whenever it is time to project. This will be impossible if you project from your bed. Furthermore, because you would be alone in this environment, there would be very few distractions for you to cope with. If your sofa has rough, uncomfortable cushions or a back alignment that irritates you, it may not be the best location to sit and relax. Try altering the cushions, adding a blanket, and moving the furniture before starting the project to make the surroundings as comfortable as possible.

If you don't want to project while lying down, you might find that projecting from your chair is a better option than sitting up. It's a terrific option because you won't fall asleep if you project from your chair during the entire. Furthermore, you will almost surely be alone in your Chair, which means no irritating traffic or people interfering with your duties.

However, in addition to its benefits, the projection of a straight chair has a number of significant disadvantages. Your body is more likely to fall into this position, causing it to be pushed out of the projection state and depositing your astral self back into your physical body before you have a chance. Otherwise, your head may flop up over your neck, depriving you of a consistent source of oxygen and potentially leading to severe breathing problems if the scenario persists for an extended amount of time.

Regardless of the mix of these three you choose, the idea is to establish a posture in which you feel safe and where your astral self may effortlessly enter and exit your body without generating any external interference or hindrance.

Start keeping a journal of your activities.

When you first begin experimenting with astral projection, it's a good idea to keep a journal of your experiences. You'll have to be quite cautious if you want to keep this going. If you have an astral experience, write down all you remember so that you can later use it to figure out patterns and improve your project skills.

1. Begin by noting the impending event's date and time. When did it take place? What did you do immediately before or after you projected? You've most likely tried it out on weekends or on vacations. Keeping track of all of this will allow you to discover the optimum time and day to generate your most effective forecasts, allowing you to select the most appropriate dates for your future forecast.
2. Before you begin, make a list of the events and conditions that transpired before your forecast. What occurred in the seconds preceding your attempt? Have you ever gotten out of bed after a particularly boozy night? If your screening was beneficial, you could try to recreate these events in the future and try

to replicate the experience while planning your next move.
3. Take detailed notes on anything that occurs throughout the screening. Keep a mental record of what transpired. Did you notice any temperature variations throughout your visit, for example? Do you get a tingling sensation throughout your body? Have you ever heard a high-pitched sound or an external voice, along with the sensation of being joined in your ascension? When you projected your thoughts, you most certainly saw other beings. All of this helps you keep control of your experiences and ensures that your projections and expectations are not influenced by destructive external forces.
4. Take note of how you were able to heal your physical body in this manner. Is there a commotion going on? Were you aware of the presence of a hostile entity, or did you manage to return safely with the assistance of a guide? If you can maintain track of all of these in the future, you'll be able to keep track of your future projections and how to channel them in order to make them more efficient, which will be really advantageous. It is not necessary to keep a logbook indefinitely. Once you've gotten used to it, you might wish to jot down some quick observations. Remember to cease practicing fully; you'll be able to do so more quickly because you'll already know what time, place, and other factors will be most conducive to your achievement at that moment.

Take control of your environment.

You can also improve your influence over your environment by employing some of the tactics described below to gain more control over your astral projections:

The implications would be severe if you were to be the one ultimately responsible for your astral self and captured as a result of your alarm's loud sound. If this is the case, your body will be taken aback, and your projection attempt will fail no matter how hard you try.

Manage the level of noise in your home: Are there any other sources of noise in your home besides your alarm? Do you have a grandfather's clock that goes off every day at 12 a.m.? What kind of noise does your air conditioner – or any other electrical equipment that you use on a regular basis – make? Take a minute to examine whether it would cause harm to a third party, regardless of how accustomed you have become to it. Instead of employing a computer system that produces interference, project your photos using a fan. If your windows are rattling, make sure they're properly sealed to prevent future problems. Make a note of everything that could interfere with your sleep or cause you to lose focus that has to be addressed ahead of time. Consider and plan for all of these scenarios ahead of time.

Prepare your friends and family: the people in your immediate surroundings may be big sources of dispute, which you should be aware of before beginning to project. Is there someone in your family that calls you every day at the same time? Is it feasible that your flatmate may knock on your door at dinnertime to inquire about special orders? Is it more frequenting for your partner to cuddle you without your permission in the middle of the night? All of these are things to consider ahead of time in order to manage your estimates properly. Reduce visibility by closing your shades or properly sealing your door, and, if possible, notify people that they will not be able to stop you at certain hours of the day. If you live in a crowded house and assume that your neighbors are unconcerned about your desires, it may be more difficult to create an environment conducive to the success of your project. Make every effort to establish conditions that allow you to spend time alone practicing projecting on a regular basis, even if only for a short period of time.

Don't forget to look after your pets. If you sleep with your favorite dog curled up next to you, your body may struggle to adjust to getting out of bed without him. Other astrologically connected entities, in addition to dogs, may cause them to respond. If this occurs, keep your pets away from the projected projection area. Keep them out of that area and lock your door to keep them out and away from your things.

Chapter 10:
Psychic Powers and Development

Develop Your Psychic Ability
Every person is born with the ability to use psychic abilities, which can be developed over time. Many people are more gifted with psychic abilities than others, and this is true for a variety of reasons. Individuals must believe that something unseen by the naked eye has occurred before they can use their psychic abilities. This test reveals that everyone has psychic energy that they can use to their advantage.

Keep a three-centimeter gap between your palms. Allow light or energy to flow through your body and into your mind by focusing your attention on your hands. When red energy is projected, it causes red energy to be generated in the palm centers. If you move your palms as if you were shooting an absolute ball, you will be able to detect an invisible object in your environment more easily.

You will notice that the ball in the center of your palm becomes firmer as you continue to add energy to it. When you bring your palms together, you will feel an invisible force between them, as if you are holding an eraser. Before you start the exercise, imagine a blue light shooting out of your plane and erasing the red ball that is currently between your hands. Then, for the rest of the exercise, imagine that your hands are still providing no energy. This is necessary to prevent your psychic energy from being continuously extracted from your body, as previously described. Didn't you seem unaffected by anything? Before you proceed, make sure you truly believe in what you're doing. There will be no progress unless and until you are confident that your mentor has the ability to unlock your psychic power abilities.

Following the discovery of psychic energy, the next step would be to practice meditation. Additional meditation is required to gain access to the invisible or psychic world. If his psychic abilities are strong enough, he should be able to see a stream of white energy moving through the air. While looking at something, repeat the phrase "color, color, color" to visualize the colors of each object.

Your ability to correctly interpret the meaning of the cards you've selected is a type of psychic ability. You will quickly develop a mental image of the cards with practice. You will gradually improve as a result of your affiliation with groups that share your psychic preferences once you are no longer required to shift cards in order to obtain the correct card or correctly interpret the card's meaning. Patience is a virtue, and one should avoid rushing through any task at all costs. You will not be able to master your psychic abilities in the time you have been given.

It is possible to have psychic abilities even if you are not particularly gifted. Even if a person's ability to access and use their subconscious is greater than that of others, psychic abilities can develop. Talented people with established psychic abilities have used their abilities to help others develop their own psychic abilities, which has had a positive impact on the world. Individuals who want to improve their psychic abilities must first improve their senses. Because of your keen observational abilities, you will notice symbolic occurrences that others will miss when you use your intuition.

Relaxation improves one's ability to tune into one's internal voice and respond to external stimuli. As a result of their constant nervousness and anxiety, many people become completely oblivious to what is going on around them. Relaxation meditation is a type of meditation that allows you to focus and concentrate on a single issue or concept for extended periods of time. The more you practice new skills, such as meditation, the more confident you will be in your ability to receive more accurate psychic readings.

Your psychic readings must be based on spiritual development that is both personally appropriate and legitimate in order to be effective. If you lack the spiritual strength or conviction to believe in spirits "outside" or in the energy that exists behind everything tangible and real, you should avoid communicating with or reading the energy of these spirits.

To develop psychic abilities, you must first strive to be your own person and live a life that allows you to follow your moral principles. Connecting with others who are interested in spirituality or psychology can help you gain a better understanding of the concept and benefit from the experiences of others who have gone through it. Spending time in a calm environment is a simple and effective method of dealing with hyperactivity. You will have a better chance of gradually adapting to your surroundings and the energy contained within them if you can consistently experience more peace each day. You must work hard to become mediums through observation and learning. Keep a close eye on what you notice and how your feelings change in response to what you notice. As you become more aware of these concepts and ideas, you will begin to see and understand them through the lens of symbols that correspond to your "sixth sense." Our actions and the energy we emit will have disastrous consequences for those in our immediate vicinity, and you will suffer the same fate. It is possible that as your awareness of the effects others have on various aspects of your life grows, you will begin to notice nonverbal or physical communications. With psychic readings, you'll begin to understand the nature of the energy you're looking for, which will manifest in a variety of ways.

You must first be aware of your own emotions and the factors that influence them in order to develop psychic abilities. The way you are treated and the way you respond to that treatment have a constant and profound influence on you. It is possible to learn to change how others perceive you by reacting differently to various events in your environment. Determine what balance means for you, and then balance your practice to increase your level of creative expression. Because a higher proportion of people have above-average levels of creativity, this is inextricably linked to how you perceive the world. To begin, it is healthy to maintain a balance in all of your activities, including sleep, eating habits, social interactions, and personal responsibilities. When you have a balanced life, you will become aware of things you previously overlooked and motivated to engage with them. When you're excited about experimenting, you'll discover new things as well as make educated guesses about what will work.

There are numerous job opportunities available. You can concentrate on whichever tool is best for you. Concentrating on the tarot cards and visualizing all of the images as a single visualization is one method for improving your psychic abilities. After combining spiritual concepts and tarot messages with a desire to relax, you'll have enough money to see the big picture. As you seek a deeper understanding of the universe and your place within it, you will come across significant information about individuals and the environment in which you live. It will take some time for you to understand how to use your psychic abilities, and you will need to relax during that time. As you continue your investigation into the psychic realm, you must accept your current life situation. Don't force yourself to accept the meaning of what you've read if you aren't ready.

It is critical to recognize that developing psychic abilities necessitates a strong physical and mental state in order to be of service to others. Pay attention when you have a strong gut feeling about something important. You may not always recognize opportunities that present themselves to you due to the options and people that come your way. You won't realize the significance of that meeting until much later in the process.

Psychokinetic and thought-control abilities, in addition to normal strength, are required. Controlling your thoughts is an important step in developing your psychic abilities and learning how to use them. Many people are hesitant to try, but once they master the fundamentals and are ready to put the techniques into regular practice, they find it to be a rejuvenating and liberating experience.

One of the many benefits of learning to control your thoughts is that you gain access to intuitive abilities that you may have overlooked, were unaware of, or had never used before. The sixth sense enhances man's psychic abilities.

As an example of imaginative thinking, asserting that you have no control over the natural processes triggered by your thoughts while they are flowing through your head is an example of imaginative thinking. Many people are afraid and anxious as a result of this situation. You can conjure up a wide range of fantastical scenarios by using your imagination. The majority of these thoughts are fleeting and insignificant, and any negative consequences you may anticipate will not occur.

As a result of this universal law, you will gain a better understanding of yourself, as well as encounter more manifestations of your personal fears in your daily life. Examining the following statement will assist you in determining whether you have psychic development potential: "The thoughts you pay the most attention to tend to manifest in your life." If this is the case, both positive and negative events in one's daily life should be affected. Right?

You can employ one or more of these strategies to assist you in developing and improving your psychic abilities. To achieve a worthwhile goal, you must put forth sufficient effort. Consider the task at hand; it will almost certainly take longer and be more difficult than you anticipated. It is also open to those who want to learn about and improve their psychic abilities.

Discover the five steps to mastering movement and realizing your psychic potential.

Daily meditation should be practiced. Over time, meditation will help you develop a stronger sixth sense, also known as your subconscious. If you don't, you'll be left with a mental image of a single, physically observable world that you can only inspect with your own eyes.

Concentrate on a few specific issues or problems that are bothering you right now. Allow your thoughts to follow their natural course. Daily repetitions of the same task train the brain. When we concentrate and focus on different areas of our brain, we can relax certain parts of our brain while simultaneously activating others. This can help us be more creative while also improving our performance and extrasensory perception (ESP). You should also keep in mind that you must stimulate your brain, which means providing it with enough stimuli to allow it to function properly.

Developing your intuition can be aided by paying attention to your inner voice. Intuition is self-acquired knowledge that has not been or will not be shared with you by another person or group of people. We occasionally have an intuitive sense of something, and it almost always turns out to be correct, leaving us all puzzled as to how it could be correct. We had to work hard to connect with our intuition before it could be unlocked; now that it is, all we have to do is learn to listen to and follow the advice of those closest to us.

When you're ready to start using your imagination for something, start by visualizing your desired outcome (but also for your own purposes). Instead, think of yourself as the only person on the planet who truly owns and possesses everything you desire.

To reap the benefits of your efforts, follow each of the aforementioned tips and give yourself a pat on the back. Allow yourself to relax and congratulate yourself on a job well done. You had accomplished your goal even before you made the conscious decision to work toward it. Because failing to do so will make it more difficult for you to discover and utilize the potential of your psychic abilities.

Making a plan to put your psychic abilities to use

Many people believe that psychics are extremely intuitive and have extrasensory perception (ESP). Psychics are used in some cultures to obtain information about the future, so their use is considered normal in those cultures. Individuals who believe in a medium are said to be able to perceive things with their senses that others cannot. The clairvoyant can assist you in clarifying your thought process.

These spiritual abilities are known as clairvoyance or psychic ability, and anyone who wants to learn how to develop and use their potential can do so. Anyone, regardless of age, social class, or educational background, has the potential to develop latent psychic powers and abilities if given the necessary information, training, determination, and commitment.

. Trusting your instincts is a good rule of thumb, in the vast majority of cases, to follow. Once we have fully utilized these resources for obtaining the things we desire in life, we will be able to maximize their potential.

Never believe anyone who claims that having psychic abilities and reaping their benefits necessitates being exceptional or gifted. The majority of people in modern society have abandoned spiritual reality in favor of material possessions, which is a depressing reality to face. As a result, these abilities have deteriorated noticeably over time. You still have a great deal of psychic power; it's just dormant and waiting to be awakened. Once you've established your psychic potential, you'll be able to tap into a wide range of useful abilities. Begin on the right foot.

Chapter 11:
Tools For an Empath's Energy Protection

True, you haven't described your aura in quite some time, have you? To keep our bodies healthy, we nourish and drink them, wash, and exercise them, brush and trim our teeth, and trim our hair and nails. We, on the other hand, almost completely disregard our bodies' most vital aspect: our auras. This is a classic case of "out of sight, out of mind," as people believe she will look after herself despite the fact that she will not.

Our auras, like our physical bodies, collect all of the dirt and debris that we come into contact with on a daily basis. The negative energy that we come into contact with affects us if these factors are not considered.

People who work in close quarters (for example, hair stylists and cosmetic therapists) are especially vulnerable to negative psychic energy accumulation. This is especially true for practitioners of energetic modalities such as massage, reiki, and reflexology.

Most healing professions do not teach students how to defend themselves against psychic attacks, and the transfer of energy between two people is rarely understood. Healers must take every precaution to keep negative psychic energy from building up in their auras.

While sleeping in at the end of the day is natural, falling behind and lacking the energy to do anything indicates that you have been the victim of a psychic attack. Protection not only allows you to better utilize your energy throughout the day, but it also aids in the capture and protection against negativity even before anxiety or stress arises.

Use your Psychic Protection ability to attract people to you.

When it comes to attracting others to you, the Fundamental Law of Attraction is unavoidably at work. You must master the art of manipulating your thoughts in order to increase your attractiveness and attract the people you want.

In other words, you need to concentrate on all of the positive things happening around you, as well as your own personal motivation to improve. You will achieve your goal if you maintain a laser-like focus on the prize and radiate positive energy to those around you. Negative energy, on the other hand, will not harm you as long as you maintain a positive attitude and stay focused."

It may appear strange that you are only now beginning to understand the concept of energy; if you are not unfamiliar with the subject, you may already have some knowledge of it; however, in order to take advantage of this once-in-a-lifetime opportunity, you must expand your knowledge of energy and psychic protection techniques.

Consider the positive events in your life to maintain a positive perspective and avoid being overwhelmed by negative thoughts. When attempting to increase your attractiveness, ensure that the energy in your surroundings is always positive. The law of attraction explains why, in general, good things happen to people who believe in it. Certain details, however, are omitted from the law.

If you are afraid of something or are having difficulty understanding something, you should address the issue(s) that are preventing you from participating in this conversation first. You will almost certainly face attacks on a much larger scale if you pursue a more elevated path and live a more positive lifestyle.

Psychic protection comes into play at this point, as it aids in preventing others from interfering with your thoughts; however, your thoughts can only be protected if the medium providing the protection is adequately trained in the situation or case at hand. Psychic Protection Spells are rarely effective at providing protection due to their simplicity.

The severity of Dupuytren's contracture (contraction of Dupuytren's fibroplasia) varies according to the intensity of the attack being fought or prevented, and those who rely on rituals and spells for psychic protection will use spells and magic to achieve their goals and protect themselves.

The most effective way to protect yourself during a psychic attack is to use a psychic shield, which can range from a bubble surrounding you to a multi-layered shield complex capable of defending you against the most powerful attacks, each of which can be classified as having a different level of intensity depending on how you describe it.

Even if you have trouble visualizing, you can make a paper shield by drawing an image of it in the center of a piece of paper on which you should draw your own image, or you can go third-dimensional and construct an object in that form to serve as your shield. Use this shield when psychic protection is required.

People who do not believe in psychic attacks, magic, or spells frequently do not take adequate precautions, which can have serious consequences. Scientists have demonstrated beyond a shadow of a doubt that the world is made of energy and that everyone emits and absorbs energy. This energy, as scientists have discovered, includes human energy. We give the other person energy while also giving them a piece of our own identity at every encounter. Psychic assassinations begin here. Even if you take adequate mental protection measures, you will frequently experience various psychic attack symptoms, whether you believe it or not.

The most extreme forms are generally considered to be black magic, voodoo, and other such spells. If you find yourself in this situation, it may be difficult to obtain psychological protection. You may require the assistance of energy workers to fully recover from the harm you have sustained. Why do you need psychic protection if you already have it? Take these psychological precautions to lessen the impact of a traumatic event and to allow your body to respond more quickly if one occurs.

To have a strong aura, you must be in control of both your soul and your physical body. The most important first step toward protecting your mental health is to improve your diet. Spending money on tobacco and alcohol exposes you to a variety of health risks as well as making you vulnerable to enemy attacks. If you eat healthily, your aura will be healthier and thus stronger. Make it a habit to use your brain for at least an hour each day.

Once you reach this level of physical well-being, attacking your aura will become significantly more difficult. Negative energy will be repelled if it comes into contact with your body.

How to Handle Negative Psychological Consequences

Avoiding any perceptions of darkness is essential for maintaining the health of your psychic energy. The most enthralling accomplishment you can achieve is to live in the present moment. The statement is, without a doubt, correct, and it is an effective defense strategy. We become preoccupied with the future, making us afraid of the unexpected. In addition, our fears deplete our aura. If the aura is weak, seizures may occur more frequently. To avoid seizures, concentrate your efforts on strengthening your aura without regard for the future. Instead, concentrate on savoring the present moment and developing a powerful aura.

Our spiritual energy is generated in the same way our physical energy is generated by our overall health. Maintaining good health is critical for living a long and healthy life as well as maintaining mental well-being. When you're feeling down, a nutritious meal can help you feel better. If you're depressed, you should feel free to read a good book or listen to soothing music to distract yourself from negative thoughts. You should not only listen to music but also immerse yourself in the spirit of singing while your psychic shields are raised. It's incredible how the music and signature work together to transport our souls, which is beneficial to our mental health.

The seemingly minor actions you can take to maintain a positive attitude will help to mitigate the negative effects of any external sources of negativity you may encounter wherever you go. Psychological defense techniques, for the most part, provide effective protection against unprovoked attacks. When a deliberate attack occurs, the attacker employs extremely dangerous techniques such as black magic, necessitating the assistance of a professional. Combating these supernatural entities on your own is extremely dangerous and may exacerbate the situation. To avoid future black magic problems, seek solutions that entail the involvement of professionals who have the necessary knowledge and training to deal with such problems.

You should also think about talking therapy. It will, however, benefit you, making it a worthwhile investment. By learning how to help your child overcome their fears, you can help strengthen their defense mechanism. You can learn techniques to protect your aura by putting in the effort and gaining knowledge.

Psychic Protection is a technique for shielding oneself against negative energy.

This rule holds true in both romantic and non-romantic relationships. Other aspects of a person's life can have an effect on their psychological health as well. Your mind has the ability to increase your attractiveness to those who already think you're attractive.

Everyone should learn the fundamentals of energy in order to protect themselves. Practicing psychic protection may help you develop greater self-confidence and strength.

The ability to protect those in your immediate vicinity is the most important factor in general. You will develop an obsession with vulnerable entities that you may have previously overlooked as a result of your newfound confidence and determination. You'll also notice your ability to deal with a wide variety of situations.

When you eliminate all negative aspects of your life, you will notice that positivity eventually triumphs over negativity. This technique is critical for appearing more appealing and manageable. The Law of Attraction is essential in understanding your own life and how it works. These are effective methods for increasing one's understanding and knowledge.

As long as you use psychic defense, you will retain control over your thoughts and actions. To put it another way, you can consider all of your ideas without focusing on any of them specifically. Avoid falling for someone who is attempting to instill negative energy in you while you are attempting to maintain a positive attitude.

Chapter 12
Dealing with an Anxious Empath

As an empath, you will never be able to change your nature. You can't change your soul's makeup, and you can't lose your advantage over other planets. Many people talk about turning empathy on and off, but this is misleading because completely turning off empathy is beyond the power of conceptualization. The most successful method has been demonstrated to be paying attention. You've come to learn how to use your empathic skill as a powerful tool for changing and transforming your life.

This is a tremendous job, and empathy must demonstrate that it is up to the task. They remove their energy from you as a result of your proximity to one another and the affection that others feel for you since your existence is full of wonder, recuperation, and veneration. This is because you agreed to it without fully comprehending it.

Even after a relationship has ended, associations or etheric ropes can be developed at various periods and for various reasons with relatives, friends, and previous sweethearts. You should seize this opportunity to break linkages!

Consider the individual with whom you are in a relationship as well as the thread that is being severed while terminating lines. After expressing kindness to the individual, say, "For the time being, I release you in kindness and light."

While there are more complicated techniques for cutting cords, this fundamental technique is both practical and straightforward. In my perspective, the more things we have to confuse, the more things become muddy. My recommendation is to keep things as simple and uncomplicated as possible.

Every night before you go to bed, ask yourself, "Do I have any relationships or connections with someone I met today?" Then, if you find something interesting, unload it and choose it.

Return a few days later to confirm that the rope has been released in double the amount. If you're unsure whether the string still exists, seek the advice of an expert. I frequently come across ropes that appear to be connected to one or more chakras or the energy field.

Because of the frequency with which your psychological body connects with the psychic array of other individuals, you are more likely to receive unpleasant thoughts from others.

Furthermore, you develop your own concerns, and some of them may compete with your most prominent ones.

For example, if you want to improve your thinking clarity, you'll need a notebook in which you'll have to write down any ideas that come to you during the next 24 hours. You'll be astonished at how difficult it is to identify your own reflection!

When your thought is certain, you may adjust to favorable vibrations and recoup, equalize, and suit your environment. Negative thoughts can stick with you for a long time, especially if associated with a particularly painful incident. Negative thoughts and desires lead to the formation of unfavorable mental patterns. They can be predicated on expectations and assumptions about the behavior of others. They will, in any event, remain buried in your mind until you have perfected the skill to focus and pay attention to your ideas.

Dread, sadness, guilt, and fury remain connected to your vitality sphere, enabling you to become increasingly receptive to these feelings. After a while, they'll ask you to draw every encounter you've ever had in your life.

These structures vibrate within you, generating a descending response on all levels of vitality, such as profound, intellectual, enthusiastic, physical, and so on. They introduce you to the vibrational patterns present in individuals, situations, and life events. It's as though you're attracting low-frequency energies to your energy field.

Examine your own life to determine whether any of these circumstances apply to you and if you are now in any situations you detest. Without you realizing it, you vibrate in resonance with them.

Your organization should monitor your vitality on a regular basis, especially if you're fatigued and melancholy, to discover if you've developed or purposefully abandoned a harmful cognitive framework.

The Chakras' Affirmation

Chakra adaptability is essential, as does regular exercise. Bathe your chakras twice a day, once in the morning and once at night, for a few minutes each time.

Make a sacred space.

Except if you're an empath, this is essential knowledge for everyone. Any place in your home can be made holy as long as you keep your independence and consider the space to be entirely self-communicating.

This might be your workshop, conference room, or simply your office, depending on your needs. This time slot must be completely dedicated to you. Make every effort not to let anyone else use this space (your kid and pets are welcome to come and leave!). It is not required to keep it indoors; instead, it can be placed outside in a lovely environment.

If you can't think of a real location, go inside your thoughts, and let go. Your mind's capabilities will astound you.

Some people imagine themselves on other worlds, in space, or on a spaceship made entirely of light energy. Others picture themselves on a beach, a desert island, or a healing sanctuary.

Smearing Yourself as Well as the Environment

Positive energy from your field of vitality is transmuted by expanding it and bringing it into contact with the earth's surface.

Maintain this exercise on a regular basis, particularly if it has increased your awareness of your emotional, mental, and physical bodies. White should be used with caution. Furthermore, if you are at home, try to smile to make your surroundings cheerful and neat.

The Interaction of Nature and Man

Nature, the most abundant source of vitality, may bring tranquility to anyone who is overwhelmed by enormous strain and pain. Empaths, I believe, are currently on the earth to help with the cleansing of adversarial energy.

People only communicate their most irritating and negative thoughts and opinions. As a result, if you are an empath, you should spend at least one hour each day alone in nature to stimulate your senses and purify your environment. If you wish to ground yourself and purify your body of negative energy, make touch with a tree.

The most effective sources of comfort and healing therapy are animals, flowers, rivers of water, and common views. Additionally, it is entirely free!

Sit with your back against a tree storage room on the ground or walk about barefoot to collect positive energy from the earth. This is known as "setting up" or "earthing," and it provides you a wonderful sense of well-being.

To protect your field of vitality, you must first recognize it.

Empaths, in my opinion, must find ways to maintain their grounding and purification on a continuous basis. In my opinion, this is the most effective type of insurance.

After clearing the heart walls, build an insurance barrier around it to safeguard it, ensure that no negative structural energies are released, and maintain a constant connection with positive energies. After clearing your Heart-Wall and building an insurance shield, all that remains is for you to build your shield.

When I deal with clients, I teach them vitality methods for maintaining a strong and healthy auric field. However, I am not as enthusiastic about the importance of insurance as I am about the importance of it.

Unless and until we allow ourselves to be exploited, we will avoid being exploited by others if we are aware of our own vitality. Your energies must be continually moving in order to execute the jobs we conduct here: digestion, transmutation, and vitality development. You'll feel sluggish and foggy if you don't do this throughout the day. This is why you keep returning to the negative aspects of your blessing and feel the need for insurance.

Working with jewels and stones increases your chances of remaining focused and aware of what is going on in your life. When it comes to defining your background, this is not an easy task.

Use critiques, art, and drawing to your advantage.

Empaths are extremely creative individuals who thrive on the opportunity to convey their abilities in a way that others can comprehend. Although they usually oppose their creative abilities when they are not feeling well, this is because crafting demands them to deal with their emotions on a regular basis, which can be difficult.

Consider using your artistic skill as a form of therapy and enthusiastic release to help you get back on track when you're feeling stuck and out of sorts.

Let your emotions be expressed through tears.

Empaths have a clever and eager physique that is pushed to cry when the situation demands it. This is because sobbing has several therapeutic effects on the body. When you cry, the vibration of your tears acts as a purifying system for your output. This is a rather regular occurrence in children.

Yoga, Tai Chi, and other energy development exercises, to name a few, can help you release tension and negative energies, purify your emanation, and transform the structure of your body and chakras.

Similarly, the vitality assignment is the most effective method for maintaining your breathing in sync with your spirit's actions.

The tenth is to take a sea salt bath.

Despite its modest size, seawater salt has amazing cleaning powers. The sea's salty air revitalizes the body. If you're feeling overwhelmed, a hot shower with sea salt will make you feel better. Regular table salt, Himalayan salt, Epsom salt, or any other salt can be used.

Chapter 13
Ways To Heal Empaths

The purpose of commencing the healing process is for you to be unable to continue on your journey. For example, if you are continually exhausted, it may be difficult for you to concentrate on assisting others. As a result, you have difficulty establishing yourself, meditating, and providing the best advice to people who are having difficulties. Aspects of your life that were once simple now appear to be difficult to achieve. You have a lot of physical sicknesses, and you don't know what's causing them, but you believe it's related to your chronic fatigue. You start to worry that something is badly wrong.

While you should always check to see if something is actually wrong, these symptoms are most likely the result of emotional exhaustion. If you have helped others in their recovery but have not prioritized your own healing or spent time removing the negative energy that has gathered in your soul, you must begin investing more time in your own recovery.

While the general public understands physical and psychological rehabilitation, emotional healing is less well-understood. When you are emotionally recovering, it is vital to pay attention to your feelings. Because of your great level of sensitivity, you and others regularly inflict emotional pain on you. In their minds, those around you are trying to help you, but they have no understanding of how your sensitivity affects your capacity to absorb and emotionally comprehend what they say. You inflict emotional misery on yourself on a regular basis as a result of your harsh words.

Recovering from Emotional Trauma

If you try to heal emotionally from an abusive background, you will almost surely spend years focused on the scars that remain. If you make a conscious effort to recover from your coworker's words, you may notice an improvement within a few days.

Whatever happens during the process of emotional healing, the first step is to acknowledge and accept it. Accept the situation as it is, as well as any residual feelings, and feel them. Consider the following scenario: you are angry at your parents and have no understanding as to why they have harmed you. If you disagree with your co-worker's assessment that you are not a diligent worker, you should accept it rather than contest it.

After accepting your sentiments, you must work through them. For example, you must understand why you feel resentful of your family. One of the most challenging components of the emotional healing process is discovering the root of your sentiments as you inquire about the best technique to use to center your emotions. Even if you are certain that you did not cause the abuse, you may question whether there was anything you could have done to warrant counseling. By asking yourself questions, you can have a greater awareness of and ability to engage with your emotions, as these inquiries allow you to access and communicate with your unconscious feelings.

These are the emotions you were having but were unaware of due to your distraction. While you evaluate your queries, you'll frequently come up with statements like "This circumstance made me so angry," when your true emotion was grief. Unconscious sentiments may be difficult to express because they are secondary emotions that come at times. They are a jumble of contradicting feelings that are difficult to classify. This is the time to employ your emotional vocabulary. Finally, you'll be able to identify and name your conscious emotion, allowing you to embark on your healing journey.

Suggestions for Emotional Reconciliation

It is tough to recuperate emotionally from a terrible occurrence. You're easily agitated and exhausted. Maintaining focus on your everyday routine will aid in your recovery. Aside from sticking to a timetable, there are a few other pieces of advice that may help you succeed in this process.

You want to do all possible to alleviate your uneasiness. Worrying makes it difficult to focus on the task at hand. You're concerned about how each stage of the healing process may affect your next steps. You begin second-guessing your every decision, obsessing over the past and worrying about the future. This makes you nervous about what might happen if you participate in your process again in the future. You're stressed out, and it's prompting you to lash out at those closest to you. As a result, you're ready to begin the healing process because all of your emotions are contributing to the stress you're experiencing right now. You have continued to grow as a result of your inability to adequately manage your emotions during the last few months. As you reflect over the last few months, you recall a number of disagreements you've had with your partner. You recall how you reacted each time they threatened to leave, claiming that it didn't matter because you were so unhappy with how things were going. You're worried that you've already alienated your sweetheart and that the damage is irreversible.

Rather than talking and sharing your discovery and practice of self-care with your partner, you become concerned when they do not return home the next day after you leave for work. As a result, your significant other will excuse themselves by claiming to be working late, attending a business meeting, or mixing with a coworker. You start to suspect your partner of cheating on you and get anxious about the matter. You bring it up in a way that makes you doubt if your partner is being entirely honest with you about what's going on.

You find it difficult to speak with your significant others as a result of your anxiety, as you are terrified of what they could say. You prepare yourself for the worst-case situation. After a few weeks, you finally find the strength to share your concerns and draw out a relationship rehabilitation strategy. Your partner eventually opens up and reveals that you have never been cheated on but that they haven't always wanted to return home with you due to the existing situations.

It's difficult to control your emotions while you're worried as your feelings are continuously shifting. You may be able to start a powerful emotional healing process by employing methods and focusing on what you can do to alleviate your worry.

Examine the most optimistic version of yourself.

Each of us has our own set of tastes. This man makes no mistakes and is always pleased with himself, always striving to achieve his best regardless of how he feels. If you visualize your faultless self, you may believe, "I'll never be so good." While it is true that perfectionism does not exist, your best self is the one you want to be every day—which is not always a negative thing.

Spend some time imagining the person you desire in your life. Make your best self more realistic and less flawless, or increase the perfection of your best self, whatever you like. You want to get a good idea of the applicant's personality. What are their counterstrategies for energy vampires? Is there a daily schedule that the individual follows?

When it comes to being your best self, the words you write represent the elements of yourself you wish to accentuate. Consider the following scenario: if you struggle to get out of bed on time every morning, your perfect self will do so effortlessly. You don't snooze when your alarm goes off; instead, you get up, get ready for the day, and have a cheerful mood throughout your awake time.

By focusing on becoming your greatest self, you can attain the mental goals you set for yourself. You could begin by describing the measures necessary to achieve these goals. To begin, get up and stand about 7:30 a.m.; however, you may get up earlier if you like. To provide yourself more time to plan, meditate, and focus on your daily tasks.

Put the past in the past.

One of the most difficult components of empathy is the desire for nostalgia. You choose to dwell on heinous incidents rather than preserve pleasant and peaceful recollections. You should do the polar opposite of what you're doing now.

The more uptight you become, the more negative your thoughts become. It serves as a reminder because the task you're working on is nearly identical to the one that caused the difficulty. You become more anxious and curious than usual about your operation. You've learned from your error and will strive not to repeat it in the future. You are well aware of your obligations. Your anxiety, on the other hand, hinders you from remembering.

Even if you're recovering and focusing on the future, you can find yourself daydreaming about the past. Avoiding reminiscing about the past is not a smart idea. Your objective is to elicit thought and then reintroduce it into your memory box. You've placed this box on a shelf and don't want it to get dust.

You are a one-of-a-kind individual.

It's simple to pretend to be someone we're not, and it's even simpler to fail. Once you have a better understanding of how your idol acts and thinks, you conduct a social media search about them. You watch their actions to learn how to copy them. Because you appreciate and respect this person, you desire to be like them. You can't think about them because you're not aware of their day-to-day challenges.

They do, however, have some of the same challenges. They are not without defects, and they, like everyone else, make mistakes. One of the most crucial pieces of advice to follow on your emotional healing journey is to avoid becoming consumed by the desire to become someone else.

Accept responsibility for your flaws and focus on your strengths. Accept responsibility for your faults and be proud of your accomplishments. Continue to be your best self while focusing on emotional recovery. You've made a nice present for yourself.

The ability to detect and comprehend one's own emotions is referred to as emotional self-awareness. Because you are aware, you may begin concentrating your attention on mending right away. Consider the following example: You're going through a rough patch in your relationship and are concerned that your lover will leave. You are well aware that the stress in your home is making you anxious. If you are aware of your emotions and can communicate them to others, you will be able to deal with them more swiftly and successfully.

Recognize your triggers.

A trigger is a life event that has an emotional influence on you. For example, if you are told that you made a mistake or that your finished product does not meet your typical standards, you may wonder why you were so anxious in the first place. Many concerns, such as "How did my parents react when I committed a mistake?" can assist you in achieving this goal. "Have I ever been fired from a job because I made a mistake?" "Do I hold myself to unrealistically high standards and strive for perfection, despite the fact that such an ideal does not exist?" After you've recognized your triggers, you can work on enhancing your self-awareness and emotional control.

You'll be bombarded with horrible memories, some of which you were not even aware of. While this may lead you down a dark alley, it is vital that you stay focused on your goal. Continue to reflect on your experiences and triggers, as well as your emotional and therapeutic objectives.

Chapter 14:
How To Cope with Stress When You're Highly Sensitive

This truth may influence your level of concern in your daily life. People who are "very sensitive" understand things more deeply than others, are better at absorbing life's intricacies, and are more receptive to both internal and external stimuli. Even something as innocuous as a provocative outfit or a vindictive companion can irritate some individuals. They will also notice when someone is compelled to accept or recognize when something terrible occurs, causing them to change their path.

Unfortunately, this increased effectiveness and awareness can lead to vigilantism, rumor, and even more worry. If you're an empath, here's how to deal with the extra worry that comes with caring for a vulnerable person or someone you care about.

You should limit your actions.

We use the term "limitations" to refer to restrictions on your capacity to connect as well as other forms of restraints. This indicates that you are gradually acquiring confidence in alerting people of your location and needs - broad ways that constrain you. For example, by leaving some wiggle room in your calendar, you can prevent feeling pressured when things go wrong, pile up, and demand additional attention. We also mean things like making sure your inbox isn't overflowing with emails.

These approaches have demonstrated where the line should be drawn. This is because it necessitates you drawing a line between your daily reality and your thoughts and feelings about it through reflective and caring activities.

As a result of contemplation practice, you may notice that you take a step back and regard your ideas, feelings, and even physical responses as entirely meaningless to your existence and "you." A handful of essential things happen when you train. To begin, you must learn to quickly calm your body, alter your pressure reaction, and return to a peaceful state. You'll also learn how to better differentiate things from things so that you're not swept away as readily when things get overwhelming. It helps to maintain balance and can also be used to build strength. Although most of this should apply to everyone, it is especially important for the overly sensitive individual.

Construct Your Own "Relaxation Zones"

As a result, your residence may become a mitigating factor, and in most cases, an undisputed one. This can be accomplished by introducing stress-relieving features such as soothing music and odor-based treatments, as well as making "downtime" available at all times.

This may also imply that you wear your comfortable ties as loosely as possible while remaining sensible. This is possible through learning about compromise systems and empathic, both of which can equip you with the tools you need to deal with future family and friend issues.

Finally, it implies that you may choose who you want in your inner circle for the rest of your life if they have proven themselves worthy, and you can distance yourself from individuals who channel, disappoint, or distract you. Furthermore, if you surround yourself with a constant flurry of adaptable and caring people when you face life's difficulties, it tends to be significantly calmer for you if you are sensitive: sensitive people require more understanding and reinforcement than others, and they are also excellent at providing it to others in similar situations.

When you have a high level of sensitivity, you are more prone to feel helpless in conditions such as insomnia, inadequate nourishment, and weariness. Resting in the nights (or wearing smooches if necessary), eating nutritious dinners, and taking care of your body, mind, and spirit in any way you can are all part of this.

Individuals who are especially sensitive have distinct obstacles. It identifies the source of your biggest concern, allowing you to enjoy a worry-free existence for the rest of your days. Pay attention to how you feel during the day and keep a pressure journal if required to measure your progress. Strengthening exercises should be included as early as possible, just as stressors should be reduced at any time.

You won't be able to change your sensitivity, but you can significantly change your lifestyle and tastes to be less affected by external stressors. This will become second nature to you sooner or later, and you will be more resistant to anxiety in general. You can only perceive benefits that are responsive to your surroundings at this time.

Techniques for coping with extremely sensitive people

According to Dr. Aron, around 15-20% of the population is extraordinarily sensitive; nonetheless, this is a feature that you have almost certainly acquired through time. HSP gathers tactile data in an unobtrusive and technologically advanced manner. The ability to identify and prepare for sounds, odors, and visual cues that other HSPs are likely to overlook is a critical component of the HSP function. The eight ways listed below will help you increase your HSP's stamina:

- Ensure that you receive enough rest. After being exposed to an irritant, your body requires time to recover. It is required to wear it for seven to eight hours per day.
- If you spend time and effort putting together a group of individuals for a variety of workouts, especially in a short period of time, you should have a backup plan in case you become overstimulated.
- Make frequent vacations a priority. HSPs require some rest to thoroughly recover and evaluate their day.
- Caffeine intake is limited or avoided. Caffeine may provide a slight lift to those who are not HSPs, but it is the rocket fuel that can lead to excessive execution and blockage in those who are.

- Alter your perspective on the situation. Develop a new strategy that will allow you to perceive the potential more clearly.
- Nature has been shown to be quite soothing for a significant percentage of HSPs.
- Take frequent pauses from your work. After incitation, your body requires time to process the incident and recover.
- Dealing with the damage caused by others, as well as dealing with occurrences that would normally not bother you, is not tough for a high-functioning personality. Limitations can help you reduce your tendency to do so.

Chapter 15:
Telepathy

When one person learns to communicate telepathically with others, they quickly learn to communicate telepathically with one another without using their five senses. Telepathy is unaffected by distance. While telepathy is considered miraculous or supernatural, it should not be because it is beyond the average person's abilities.

There are numerous types of telepathy, as well as subcategories within each type. This is the very first instance of people communicating their emotions through the medium of language. These sensations are distinct and extremely sensitive, despite the fact that they are frequently felt in the recipient's solar plexus. Animal empathy, a lesser-known but more common form of telepathy, is possible for both humans and animals. People are more likely to form an emotional telepathic connection when they are in direct physical contact with one another or share an aura. In the field of telepathy, spontaneous telepathy refers to the ability to read another person's thoughts without their knowledge or effort, and it is one of the most basic and primitive forms of telepathy that anyone can experience.

The exchange of brief phrases, such as words or phrases, between two people's thoughts is the third type of telepathy. Suppressing unwanted thoughts and emotions is well known to aid in the healing process. Telepathic communication may be disrupted in the event of a message transfer attempt. Even if communication is potentially dangerous, it is preferable if it is permitted.

When large groups of people communicate, a phenomenon known as mass telepathy occurs. This is your emotional state in relation to a specific location or town. You've almost certainly been accepting of this incredible telepathy the entire time. Telepathy on a large scale occurs in both the workplace and in one's personal life. Being aware of your surroundings allows you to distinguish between situations that make you feel alienated and those that make you feel uneasy.

Meditation, hypnosis, binaural beats, and a variety of other mind-calming techniques can all be used to aid in the development of telepathy. When the mind is calm and still, it is easier to receive and send telepathic communications. You can eliminate all mental and static noise from a situation by tuning your radio to a specific channel. This is analogous to tuning a radio station to a specific frequency.

When we recognize that we are constantly transmitting and receiving information but are unaware of it, the law of attraction becomes more apparent. Furthermore, when we are consumed by relationships and fear, we unintentionally alienate those who are looking for a positive and healthy relationship. Why do men keep telling you that once you marry, women will constantly be vying for your attention? Do you know why they say this? The women recognize the gesture as an act of kindness and a point of connection between them.

It is critical for him to maintain a positive attitude toward the people he meets and toward his own thoughts in general by constantly communicating with them via telepathy.

Telepathic Communication Between Two People's Minds

Almost everyone is capable of telepathy. Telepathy is defined as the transmission of information without the use of physical senses such as vision, hearing, or touch.

Telepathy is a term that refers to the receiving and transmitting of thoughts from minds that are not dependent on sensory outcomes or are unaffected by the sensory world. It refers to the reception and transmission of thoughts by minds that are not sensory-dependent. For those interested in learning more, know that your brain's strength lies in its ability to read minds and develop intuition through the use of your brain's power, not your hearing, sight, or feeling.

We've all tried to "read someone's mind," either to laugh at the absurdity or as a simple expression of happiness. What you have witnessed is a much cruder form of telepathy, but it is still a highly advanced form. Despite the fact that the subconscious screen is only a small window into your brain's and mind's incredible power, it is sufficient to accomplish anything you set your mind to. What would your life be like if you had the ability to communicate through telepathy?

Telepathy, like any other skill, can be learned, but it must be practiced in order to be effective. To use telepathy effectively, you must first gain access to your subconscious, also known as your subconscious mind. Because you can concentrate solely on communicating telepathically with the person with whom you wish to communicate, your chances of mastering this skill improve. Binaural Mp3 beats and isochoric tones would be used to increase the effectiveness of this straightforward and disciplined approach.

Using these telepathy techniques, you can find out if you have telepathy or not.

If you are a beginner or an amateur, your first attempts should take no more than 15 minutes. Allow your initial failures to affect you and make you feel bad about yourself. When attempting telepathic communication, it is important to maintain a focused and clear mental energy.

When it comes to telepathy and seawater, a small difference in communication channels can make a big difference. Make the most of your time in the ocean by swimming as frequently as possible or by keeping bottles of bottled seawater on hand.

Before attempting to capture the image, ensure that you are physically fit and arrange your assets in a sequence with one or more other assets as well as a numerical value, picture, or location.

See yourself in a calm, peaceful, and welcoming environment for a moment. It makes no difference what you want to create as long as you are completely at ease and comfortable in your surroundings. Visualize yourself walking through this area in your mind for a moment. Allow the images to appear after that. Allow it to happen on its own. Rather than attempting to communicate with the person in front of you telepathically, try visualizing them in your mind's eye. You should thoroughly read and comprehend the information provided to you, as you will be sending and receiving direct communication in this situation. When you first start practicing telepathy, you may notice physical sensations near your solar plexus.

All meditation techniques involve rewiring the brain and mind in such a way that these skills and abilities become possible. Simply listening to mp3 beats and isochoric tones can train your brain to operate at that frequency and state, allowing you to perform these tasks.

To increase the likelihood of people communicating telepathically, this treatment induces an ideal mental state conducive to telepathy, in which all other thoughts and distractions are blocked, and the mind is placed in an alpha brain state. Higher thoughts, spiritual epiphanies, and "Eureka" moments are all common in the alpha state, as are sudden "Aha!" moments. Because you are in an Alpha state, you can devote your full attention to developing your psychic abilities without being distracted by outside influences or thoughts. It is possible to facilitate mental exercises by creating an ideal environment.

Furthermore, they are easy to find. Thought transference is the other technique. Anyone with the ability to develop telepathy can learn it. Many of you have heard the term "telepathy," which translates to "mind-reading." For those who are unfamiliar with the concept, here's a quick explanation. While understanding another person's thought process without speaking to them is possible, telepathy is a completely different phenomenon. Certain people have the ability to understand what others are thinking without having to directly communicate with them. This is referred to as nonverbal communication. Scientists believe that because people's frequency levels are similar, their thoughts are capable of transmitting frequencies through the air from one person to another.

When there is no verbal communication, it can be useful to gain insight into someone's thought process. So far, we've discovered some helpful telepathy software. Telepathy is only possible when the mind is calm, which is not always the case. This program is easy to obtain and pay for, as well as reasonably priced.

Before one can comprehend one's own thought processes, one must be aware of them. This software is great for both mental training and relaxation. Effective mind-to-mind communication requires only a narrow frequency range. This software provides a step-by-step guide to increasing the efficiency of your brain in these frequency ranges.

This computer program contains a number of recording rhythms that both energize and completely relax the brain. As a result, the brain focuses solely on a few beats, ignoring everything else. Cerebral telepathy greatly expands your options. The brain must be relaxed in order to properly absorb frequency signals.

Interpersonal relationships are greatly influenced by telepathic communication. A husband can sometimes figure out what his wife is thinking even if she does not express it directly to him. He gives his wife exactly what she wants and acts in a way that she values. It's impossible not to be envious of this woman because she's married to a man who can read her mind and knows exactly what she's thinking without her saying anything. This ability is derived from telepathy, a type of mind reading. Improve your interpersonal relationships by honing your telepathic abilities.

Nobody, including you, possesses telepathic abilities. Sometimes intuition is referred to as instinct, and other times it is simply referred to as intuition. The concept, on the other hand, remains constant. With dedicated training and the development of telepathy abilities, anyone can become an expert.

Telepathy is a natural human ability that can be utilized while under hypnosis. On a daily basis, people enter and exit unconscious altered states of mind, but they are completely unaware of it.

What if you were constantly switching between states of consciousness throughout the day, multiple times a day? When you become aware that you are dreaming when you awaken, whether you are preoccupied with a television show or a movie or simply immersed in what you are reading, you can reflect deeply on your thoughts.

When it comes to our survival in a world where our thoughts and intuitions are almost always present, the instincts of any species motivated by the desire to survive defines our lives.

In order to optimize neural pathways in your brain, your body is designed to cycle through different stages of sleep.

These rhythms appear to repeat every ninety minutes. People like that exist to give your mind a break from the numerous tasks you must complete throughout the day. They allow your mind to process and assimilate their experiences, allowing you to access them later.

To achieve these periods of mental calm, scientists believe that entering the REM sleep cycle is just as important as exiting the REM sleep cycle. If you do not get enough of these natural sleep cycles, you may find yourself unable to complete daily tasks. This superior state of mind is defined by the presence of human telepathy while in a trance state that can be considered natural hypnosis.

As a result of its allure, it has attracted some distractions, such as unproven telepathy myths and outright accusations that it is terrible.

Abusing something has negative or long-term consequences for the abuser; it should go without saying. Only those who are aware of their actions and choose to participate in them will face negative consequences. When a rational statement is violated, such as the laws of nature, disciplinary action must be taken. Success necessitates the ability to be positive and helpful, as well as the ability to use telepathy for the benefit of others at all times.

This ability enables you to connect your mind and body in a unique and valuable way. It enables you to perform incredible feats with minimal effort. Human telepathy allows you to use your body's natural ability to request and effect change. It is a form of hypnosis or guided imagery that allows you to access your body's natural ability to request and effect change. When done in conjunction with a higher power, this is referred to as a prayer in many cultures.

A human-to-human telepathic connection, like guided imagery, is used to help others heal and to improve your overall well-being, as well as to boost your brain's power. True because it has been demonstrated that learning in an abstract state of mind allows you to learn faster and more effectively, and you are more likely to remember what you have learned. Consistent and controlled use of these trance states can help you achieve mental capacities you never imagined possible.

Psychometry

The use of psychic abilities to gain psychic access to the past of an object by touching or holding it against one's forehead is known as psychometry. Psychometry practice with letters can make the process much easier. Written communication is advantageous because it allows for the rapid development of telepathy abilities through the provision of immediate feedback. Consider how others will perceive you if they notice a letter scribbled across your brow. As you continue reading, you'll notice that you're developing opinions about the letter's author, the setting in which it was written, and the letter's content.

It's an exciting story about a letter written from France to the United States that exemplifies the time's values, history, and society. Every time the letter was sent, the address was changed. It had been a perplexing circumstance. He had arrived at his destination after a long journey and was now delivering the letter to a young Indian girl with the gift of psychometry. Her descriptions of the locations mentioned in the letter, as well as the people and situations she encountered along the way, were meticulous.

Telepathy Psychometry's effectiveness is object-dependent; typically, the best results are obtained when an object has previously had frequent contact with a specific individual. When performing psychometry, it is beneficial to have personal items on hand, such as jewelry, clothing, hair, and other personal belongings. Minerals and metals are more difficult to obtain than other commodities due to their unreliability. Certain people can see an item's entire history, including who it has been linked to, as well as comprehend its unique characteristics. Psychometrists are individuals who are solely concerned with their own future. When practicing or testing, strive for a diverse application and testing of psychometry. The majority of people are unable to see into the future or the past, and they are also unable to read and comprehend the entire letter. The majority of experts in their field practice psychometry or reading another person's thoughts. Once you've identified your psychometrics niche, you can devote the majority of your time and effort to developing it.

If you work with an item after it has been handled by several people, you run the risk of developing an incorrect impression of it. There are currently no established protocols governing the use of psychometric telepathy. Individuals can gradually improve their psychic abilities by adhering to a few basic guidelines. The specifics are as follows: This is advantageous for a student of psychometry. Develop an understanding of how to use psychometrics so that you can quickly assess your performance

Increasing one's understanding of how to use the Telepathy ability

Individuals will communicate using one or more of their five senses. Despite the fact that we all have a sixth sense, the vast majority of us choose to disregard it. Before you can use your sixth sense, you must first master the fundamentals of telepathy.

There are many different interpretations, skeptics, and years of practice when it comes to telepathy. For the time being, we'll limit our discussion to the fundamentals of the technique. Once you've mastered the fundamentals, it'll only be a matter of time before you're ready to try more advanced techniques.

Kinesics is the most basic form of telepathy for learning and is a nonverbal mode of communication used to convey information. The most well-known nonverbal communication technique is kinesics. When twins are suspected of anticipating what their peers will say before they have finished speaking, it is referred to as Kinesics. People criticize this nonverbal form of communication because it is performed, which is why it is controversial. Despite the fact that they must have telepathy, they are very familiar with one another.

Concrete thought transmission is a higher level of telepathy than simple thought transmission. This app's functionality refers to the exchange of objects or symbols between two people. To begin telepathic communication, you must first notify a friend who will receive the telepathic message. It is critical for both individuals to maintain a direct line of sight with the beam as it passes from one to the other. If you had focused equally on both, your friend should have been able to verbalize the data he sent. The continued application will aid in the mastery and development of this technique.

To receive a message effectively, you must give it your undivided attention. It is preferable to receive your messages rather than converse with a friend. If you ask a friend to send you a color that is completely focused on it, you will gain a better understanding of the color. Once you've grasped the message, you'll be able to see and understand everything.

The process of establishing telepathy is straightforward.

Following these simple guidelines will help you improve your telepathic abilities.

Believe in the possibility of communicating with others through telepathy.

Regardless, make a concerted effort to keep your thoughts about whether or not someone has telepathic abilities private from yourself and others. When you believe something is impossible, your mind and intuition collaborate to ensure you're correct (unless your mind is feeling bad, of course, in which case it will try to disprove it).

Find a sparring partner to practice with.

I strongly recommend that you find another person in your area who is interested in honing their mental abilities as a telepath and shares your enthusiasm for doing so! If this is not an option, look for a telepathy forum online and look for a partner there. Working with a telepathy collaborator will benefit you in a variety of ways, including giving you the massive amount of encouragement you'll need to find your creative stride.

Alternatively, you can complete the task yourself if you prefer.

Telepathy practice does not necessitate the use of a telepathic device. For instance, you could deal the cards face down and then flip them over to see if you've gained any new abilities. There are numerous telepathy downloads available to assist you in improving your telepathy skills and abilities.

Even if you're just starting out, this will put you under a lot of pressure, so keep it short and sweet. Furthermore, having a high level of energy before beginning is essential; some light exercise will help.

Learn how to unwind and relax.

An increased effort will make the task more difficult to complete while de-stressing. When you first begin studying telepathy, you may not be as skilled as you would like. The Sedona Method may be useful if you need extra help relaxing. This technique will assist you in relaxing in a short period of time.

Telepathy can be used in dreams.

When you are awake, you are not limited to using telepathy only while sleeping. Even if you don't believe you'll be able to control your dreams, starting to record them as soon as you wake up is a good place to start.

You will improve your ability to recall your dreams. When you begin dreaming telepathically, you will be inundated with thoughts from your deceased loved ones on the other side of the world.

Chapter 16:
Clairvoyance

They can grow normally with the assistance of clairvoyant forces. Many people believe that deep thought has numerous benefits for the mind, body, and soul, as well as for one's personal financial situation. Spending a few minutes each day alone with your thoughts and feelings can help you quiet your mind and calm your nerves. Include an air supply system as well. Choose the breathing technique that feels the most natural to you. Incense and candles can also enhance the overall experience.

Another great tip for those looking to improve their clairvoyant abilities is to keep constant track of them. Write down everything you see, hear, and feel while you're thinking about it. Make a mental note of your emotions in order to keep them safe. Think about each image that comes to mind, and you might discover that you have a long-term impact on the world. To progress through the clairvoyant force's levels, you must be able to clearly visualize events, people, and places within yourself. On a regular basis, reverse your statements. This should happen after you've taken some time to consider how your work relates to genuine moments in your life.

When you use your intuition, you can access all of your faculties. Maintain a regular awareness of the people who are important to you, and then try to see them "through" rather than "at" them. Consider how the earth encompasses everything and how it reflects the thoughts and feelings of those who inhabit it. The more attentive you are, the less complicated things appear.

Learning to communicate with spirits and becoming a clairvoyant medium can be time-consuming and exhausting. Keeping a diary allows you to regularly develop your sixth sense, also known as clairvoyance, reflect, and monitor your emotions and images. Our soul guides, angelic helpers, and departed friends and family members rarely appear as images or contemplations that can be interpreted as soul signs.

The more clairvoyant abilities you develop, the better you will become at detecting these unusual situations.

The ability to stimulate psychic abilities and mystical experiences in oneself or others.

The term "mystic" has taken the work out of mysticism, making it more difficult to accept; the concept of an otherworldly "homecoming" is overly optimistic. A clairvoyant is someone who has natural spiritual abilities and uses them to receive and transmit God's messages for the benefit of others. This is possible at a higher vibration level and in a more intense state than previously. A spiritualist or prophet is frequently endowed with a natural blessing or gift as a result of their profession. It is observed to emerge and grow over time when "typical" conditions are met. Whatever happens, the mystic gains vital knowledge about an extraordinary otherworldly plane of existence.

Fortunately, we have a diverse set of capabilities and resources at our disposal. Individuals with a completely open mind can acquire and use any of these assets to achieve their objectives. The blessings are perceived in addition to or as a result of the five known faculties, which include, among other things, location, sound, taste, touch, and smell, and there are several references to intuition or extrasensory perception throughout the book (ESP). As a person gets closer to their essence and heavenly potential, heavenly or otherworldly blessings begin to flow into their life. Furthermore, a more global perspective is required to aid in the enrichment process. To avoid getting the heebie-jeebies, I recommend that you overcome any occult-related fears you may have. Because you're worried about it, you almost never put your good fortune to good use. We must use these wonderful tools if we are to have the same level of devotion to Jesus as he did. It's common knowledge that my father would be unconcerned if you used His resources, so let's look at some of the benefits.

Extrasensory perception is the ability to perceive objects that are not visible to the naked eye.

Clairvoyance, also known as clear vision, is the ability to see into one's own heart. This enables you to examine images from someone else's life in order to better understand their personality. Depending on their level of extrasensory development, extrasensory individuals may perceive things through their physical or profound senses (eyes, messengers, spirits, and images from the otherworldly realm), or they may see holy messengers, spirits, and various scenes from the otherworldly realm. This blessing may appear in dreams or during waking hours if the third eye (or sixth chakra) is clear and open. God provides us with internal vision today, just as He did for the prophets of old.

Clairaudience
Another manifestation of psychic blessing is clairaudience, which occurs when people are gifted with messages from other realms through their hearing. People with this ability are more likely to receive messages from the soul and/or their own minds. Saint Joan of Arc bestowed her blessing on me when she presented this to me.

Clairsentience
Psychometry, also known as clairsentience, is the ability to communicate with an object and elicit detailed information about its previous owner. This ability is only possessed by a small number of people. This blessing bestows upon you the ability to predict events in other people's lives before they occur, similar to having a premonition.

Clairempathy
It is possible to feel another person's emotions, torment, or needs as a result of one's compassion. When a global disaster or a personal tragedy strikes close by, those who have been blessed with this blessing may find themselves recharging their batteries and stepping into the shoes of another. If you're experiencing unexplained pain or strange feelings, it's possible that you've consumed the vitality of another person. Those

with this ability will gain a better understanding of the magnitude of limitations if they can define them.

Clairgustance
The ability to receive information from the transcendent domain through the sense of taste is referred to as "clairgustance." You might be given a chance to try something new or interact with someone you've never met before.

Clairscent
Individuals with the Clairscent smell ability can tell the difference between scents from their own domain and scents from other domains. A clear taste gift, also known as clairgustance, is similar to an endowment. While kneeling in worship, I've been inhaling a variety of incredible scents I've never experienced before. Heaven's kingdom is contained within your nostrils.

Chapter 17:
Psychic Ability and Spirituality

The ability to communicate with vitality threads that exist above the 'typical' level of physical reality is defined as psychic capacity. Associating with explicit vitality threads suggests the possibility of reading future and past events, learning about the other world, and resurrecting the dead, to name a few. For the better part of a century, the term "psychic" has been used to describe a wide range of abilities and capacities that are now thought to have a spiritual or supernatural component. To avoid confusion, these abilities should be classified as 'correspondence' development.

When we realize how inextricably linked the two concepts are, it becomes much easier to comprehend the concept of 'otherworldliness.' It's a common occurrence that will almost certainly reoccur in the future. Religious doctrine defines souls as having a variety of meanings that vary by religion and belief, but the fundamental meaning remains the same. The most precise correspondence is always that which is sent as soon as possible. It's like having a conversation with someone. Instead of storing data for later use, being present and conversing authentically will produce more accurate results.

The ability to manifest psychic abilities is one of the many features of our extensive collection of specialized equipment. There was no way to connect with and embrace the soul or other emotional substances present prior to the development of psychic abilities. The ability to communicate deeply is not implied by psychic ability alone. In order to have a profound correspondence, there must be an expectation of association. The reader is then aided in comprehending and becoming more familiar with the material through the use of resources and language of association.

To establish a psychic connection with the soul, one must be aware of one's selflessness. While explicit planes and measurements are observed, assistance and preservatives are used to keep procedures open and free of impediments. While some people may be able to accept the limitless soul if they are mentally prepared, the vast majority of people will find it difficult to surrender to limitless awareness. Because the most complete representation of the mind (the human brain) is solid and concrete, this is the case. As we become more established or progressive, these examples become more ingrained in our minds. Dedicated practice, nuance, and a strong commitment to practicing self-dominance are all required for success.

We must reject the cutting-edge world's proclivity to promote semantic dependency. Finally, semantics and words imply that words and ideas are meant to convey true meaning and comprehension. In this location, a person's psychic ability can open up a world of possibilities. We can see things to their very core because of our psychic abilities. These life force tangles pull us down their paths while steering us away from ours. What if the channel is more grounded and clearer than our physical body? This becomes our line of inquiry as we approach the soul, the association, and the correspondence.

A "psychic" person is capable of perceiving and identifying information that others cannot see or feel. Extrasensory Perception (ESP) differentiates those who possess it from those who do not. Psychics come in all shapes and sizes. Certain people have an intuitive sense of the air around them; others can read other people's minds, and still, others can pass on information to those who stay with them. According to some psychics, the majority of people have an innate psychic ability, also known as a "gut feeling." The majority of psychic abilities are based on innate mindfulness, which usually remains dormant until a person devotes significant time and effort to cultivating and refining it.

While the vast majority of psychics are born with the ability, there is growing evidence that it can be taught. Studying the various books available and becoming familiar with the various nuances of being a psychic will greatly aid in understanding the subject's nuances. Taking a psychic test that assesses a person's ability to perceive things other than their own self-evident truths can reveal how far a person's ability to perceive things other than their own self-evident truths can be extended.

Once a person's psychic abilities are discovered, there are numerous methods for honing and developing them to the point where they can be recognized as a distinct psychic ability. While mental capacity is important, it must be used in conjunction with focus and concentration in order to be effective. Before you can fully develop your psychic abilities in any other area of your life, you must first master these two fundamentals. A psychic is someone who has been exposed to a wide range of previously unknown elements. Human survival and development necessitate extreme emotional and sentimental endurance, as well as the ability to perceive without becoming meditative. This is significant because it demonstrates their ability to think strategically and comprehensively.

Another way to improve one's mental abilities is to maintain a positive outlook on life. This energy has an incredible ability to broaden one's horizons and expose oneself to an infinite number of possibilities. It is critical for the psychic to be unrestrained. Stress impairs a person's mental abilities and causes them to overlook a person's full or genuine comprehension. The term "third eye" refers to a type of extrasensory awareness that some people possess. By calming your mind and body, you can strengthen your third eye, increasing your chances of success as a psychic.

It's difficult to convey the concept of psychic mindfulness in a single illustration. Individuals will perceive the world of their existential encounters through a variety of actions, the extent to which their vitality detecting and influencing abilities develop. As a result, psychic abilities manifest in a variety of ways. This is because being is both malleable and synergistic.

People go through a series of stages of criticism in their daily lives on a physiological level. On a daily basis, real-world examples of the effectiveness of genuine nature protection can be found in a large number of input circles. To remove these impediments from the very core of one's being, one must first learn how to remove them. As a result, the creative specifications become more open, and any impediments to maximum articulation are removed.

Last but not least, the topic of total awareness is being widely discussed. At this level, psychic abilities and physical presence are used in ways that are far beyond what is normal or fanciful on a daily basis. This does not rule out the possibility that extrasensory perception and awareness of vital energy in other dimensions serves a purpose. We can use our abilities more effectively if we maintain a calm and educated demeanor. This entails tearing down both self-deluded examples of resistance and meaningless links that undermine the concept of unity alone.

Remote surveys are frequently thought to be concerned with information and data collection. There are two ways to incorporate psychic mindfulness into your life: In one case, it is used as a strict standard to ensure the accuracy of data collected for specific purposes. The fundamental premise of traditional remote review is the collection of precise data for clearly defined targets and objectives.

Unlike remote survey strategies, these do not involve the development or enhancement of the observer's conscious mindfulness. Under predetermined conditions, the machine operated in an overly fixed state and produced predictable results. While almost anyone can do so, focusing more on self-development results in little to no improvement in overall capability.

Remote survey procedures are limited by the fact that they are typically carried out from the incorrect vantage point. Remote review is seen as a way for those who have not yet established a connection to data "outside of themselves" to gain access to "external" data.

As you progress to higher levels of conscious mindfulness, you will recognize that this belief is false. Everything in the universe is intertwined in a healthy whole and exists in various components of a fully functioning, vibrantly alive state. The measurements become more complex and interconnected as they progress towards the eye or core of internal stillness at the center of all room time. Everything comes from the still void of infinite possibility that surrounds us.

We can see how this is possible when we consider the possibility of remote surveying. Everything has a core, and that core is a carbon copy of everything before it. Remote review strategies function in this manner because they guide the individual toward self-awareness. A successful psychic preparation method allows the individual to enter this cycle of constant communication and emerge re-energized and reconnected to their true self.

Chapter 18
Reiki Healing

Reiki treatment, as is clear, has a direct effect on stress levels and tension release in the body. It can also boost the effectiveness of the body's natural healing systems.

The question then becomes, how does Reiki aid in body healing while also relieving stress? The answer to this query remains an enigma. Reiki's impact, on the other hand, has been the topic of an increasing number of research. Current studies indicate that it has a calming effect on the heart, blood pressure, and the generation of stress hormones. Despite the fact that the benefits of Reiki have been demonstrated, we can only conjecture on what causes them and how they are produced. Reiki affects us on many levels, and the benefits are frequently felt immediately. This illustrates that Reiki is a sophisticated process that affects many different body systems at once. Following the commencement of a stressful situation, the body transitions from a stressed state (also known as combat or flight mode) to a relaxed state in which it is ready to heal itself, a process known as parasympathy. Many scientists believe that this transformation occurs unknowingly in a region known as the biofield, which also happens to be the location of the shift.

What does the organic field's name mean?

The "biofield" is the electromagnetic field that surrounds the physical body. Medical research has embraced the term to describe the region's vibrating energy field. There is no method to explore the biofield because current technology has not been able to establish its presence. As previously said, traditional and indigenous civilizations have recognized this energy biofield for thousands of years and have always regarded it as a crucial component of their people's health and well-being. It was anticipated that disrupting this biofield would result in a loss of homeostasis and the onset of illness. As a result, just because science hasn't advanced far enough to explore this occurrence doesn't mean it should be rejected.

Vibration is utilized to repair the mind and body in a variety of traditional healing modalities, including shamanic healing. This includes humming and ceremonial drumming, as well as singing and singing. This has motivated musicians to compose music with the express purpose of raising or lowering people's energy levels to the desired level. Weightless was written by Marconi Union to assist those who are concerned. Music has been shown to reduce stress levels by up to 60% when listened to with one's eyes closed. As a result of listening to the song, you may notice a change in vibratory frequency as your body's natural rhythm realigns. Others believe Reiki's healing advantages stem from a similar vibrational mechanism that promotes body coherence while decreasing body discord. Another theory is that the energy vibrations transmitted to the recipient are contained in the hands of a Reiki practitioner.

Depending on their present state of health, the client's consciousness may be adjusted to coincide with the healing power they believe is the key to their well-being. The purpose of many therapies is to restore the patient's biofields' equilibrium. Reiki is regarded as one of the gentlest therapies available because it employs vibration rather than physical manipulation or even light force. Reiki practitioners also assert that energy functions on a field known as the united field rather than the biofield.

Reiki has a number of advantages over other forms of therapy. According to the National Center for Complementary and Integrative Health, Reiki is a complementary medical method that enhances proven treatments by harnessing energy that science has not yet identified. The majority of energy healing treatments are founded on the notion that humans are surrounded by and exist within a specific form of energy. Many Reiki practitioners believe that Reiki is fundamentally different from most other energy therapies and, as previously said, is more akin to meditation. Numerous energy healing methods use specialized procedures to get access to a person's biological field in order to affect changes; Reiki, on the other hand, does not attempt to diagnose problems or change the energy field on purpose. When the energy affects them, they become more submissive. Reiki, by definition, is a somewhat passive kind of energy healing. The practitioner's hand remains motionless for the majority of the treatment. This only happens when they switch hand positions. A Reiki practitioner is a neutral person who does not attempt to affect or influence the person receiving treatment's energy field. Rather than striving to harness Reiki energy, a Reiki practitioner merely rests his body.

You can support yourself if you have an open wound or a burn that has to be treated by placing your hands directly above your torso. In response to a client's need for balance in specific areas of life, the practitioner's energy flows freely. While the practitioner's technique is fundamentally the same for each session, each treatment is tailored to the client's individual needs. A full Reiki session is suggested, but certain regions of the body can be handled in a shorter session. Even a few minutes of Reiki can make a tremendous difference in stressful situations.

Reiki is administered during the cure session.

Reiki sessions are not standardized, do not have a set length, and do not require precise adherence to a system to be effective. Anyone who has completed the relevant training can execute this duty. The individual in question could be a professional, but they could also be a doctor, a friend or family member, or even you! Furthermore, the atmosphere is not characteristic of Reiki. Reiki is most effective in a calm environment, although it can be delivered anywhere, regardless of what is going on in the immediate surroundings or with the person receiving it. It is not uncommon for a few moments of Reiki to become an emergency. It is typically administered immediately following an injury, as well as during and after surgery.

To ensure the greatest possible experience, conduct some preliminary research before selecting a practitioner with whom you feel comfortable. Choose if you want Reiki from a friend or from a stranger. This can help you bond if you have a companion with whom you entirely feel comfortable. If you are naturally uneasy around foreigners, you may choose to employ an expert with more experience. Meet with your practitioner ahead of time, if possible, to get a sense of who she is and what to expect from the session. Throughout your search, look for a practitioner who describes the procedure in detail and specifies how they intend to prepare the session. While every Reiki session is different, knowing what to expect before entering the room is usually beneficial.

How is the system configured?

The optimal environment for you is one in which you feel comfortable with yourself and your surroundings. When they pay visits to your house, they usually carry a lot of information on how to create the best setting. Practitioners frequently utilize calming music and ambient sounds to assist clients relax during sessions

Professional practitioners can treat patients for up to 90 minutes at a time. The great majority of Reiki treatments fall somewhere in the middle.

Reiki is generally administered as gentle touches with the practitioner's hands placed at various points on the body. The individual's head, as well as the front and back of the torso, are included. A practitioner should not touch or be obtrusive in his or her patient's personal parts. Additional implantation on damaged physiological components, such as the arm, may be required as needed. If you have a tight grip on the device, the practitioner may also hold your hands directly above the area of discomfort.

How would you summarize your overall impressions of the experience?

Reiki is a highly individual experience. Typically, the changes are small and are not immediately evident to the recipient. Many people describe experiencing a variety of comparable sensations and experiences during Reiki therapy. Some people have described feeling a throbbing sensation in the area where the practitioner's hands are positioned as energy waves move through the body. Several folks have mentioned how at ease they felt during the talk. According to one study, participants described floating in another dimension of awareness while remaining entirely aware of and drawn to their surroundings. Others claimed to have entered a deep level of meditation as a result of the event, while others believed it was very theatrical.

While some people may dislike their first Reiki treatment, the vast majority report feeling terrific afterward. The most common outcome is a profound sense of relaxation and immediate tension relief.

Reiki's benefits accumulate over time, and even people who don't feel anything at first describe more strong sensations as their sessions progress. In addition to the immediate impacts of Reiki, you may notice more beneficial changes in your life in the days following your session. Improved digestion, increased attention, and deeper sleep is just a few of the benefits.

Chapter 19
Lucid Dreaming

Lucid dreams occur when the dreamer is aware of the events taking place in the dream. The individual has already left his or her body during the lucid dream.

Lucid dreams, often known as consciousness while dreaming, are one of the most fascinating varieties of sleep. Because dreams are so vivid, many people feel that certain events in their dreams are reenacted in their waking lives. Lucidity in dreams is a state of consciousness that almost all dreamers have experienced at some point in their life. If, on the other hand, you can communicate clearly in your dreams, you may rewrite them and lead them in any way you like. When you reinterpret the dream, you regain entire control of your current actions and sensations. Many people have had dreams that were lucid at some point in their lives, but most don't realize it.

To characterize these types of experiences, the term "lucid dreaming" was recently coined. The ability to become aware of one's surroundings while dreaming is the core definition of lucid dreaming. After that, you'll be able to influence and modify what happens in your dreams. If you master this skill, you will be able to achieve magical feats that even Harry Potter couldn't, such as controlling your own fate and becoming the hero of your own story. True lucid dreaming, on the other hand, is still rather rare. Many people just have to cope with it once and never learn to properly control their sleep. This is because people are unable to sustain mental awareness when dreaming. When you sleep, you have no conscious control over anything. You will be accommodated in an ever-changing cycle of events.

When you have lucid dreams, you are in a state of sleep consciousness that allows you to perform great feats in real life. They enable you to visualize past events and plan for the future. One of the most beneficial parts of lucid dreaming is the ability to revisit crucial periods in your life. If you have a definitive performance, you can imagine it flawlessly every time before the actual event happens. You can practice relaxing and letting go of stress and tension by becoming aware of your dreams and sleep prior to an important event. As a result, you'll be motivated and confident on the day of the event, which is a major advantage. Another significant benefit of lucid dreaming is the capacity to travel to many places of the world. You can begin building your dream home, relocate to any region, and explore the area.

You can utilize your imagination before waking up to create exciting dreams and situations that allow you to explore and discover new worlds. Before you begin training, ensure that you and your teammates understand each other and that you have established your own goals for how you will use them in the future.

This knowledge will help you achieve in all facets of your life by providing you with new perspectives on the past and the future. Stress and exhaustion are common causes of lucid dreams. According to research, the presence of significant amounts of carbon dioxide in your bloodstream is the major cause of this mental state. As a result of its use, this stimulant induces the breakdown of energy-producing substances in the brain, such as adrenaline and serotonin.

Your body produces a large number of sleep-related hormones, which contribute to this mental state. Dopamine, for example, is usually associated with the appearance of vivid and intense sleeping dreams. If you're having difficulties sleeping because of anxiety, you're more likely to have lucid dreams. The ability to be aware of your dreams without becoming fully awake and aware of your surroundings is a critical talent for experiencing clear dreams. Improve your capacity to focus completely on one memory or thought at a time. The goal is to learn how to stay awake throughout your dreams and to focus your sleep on a certain image or thought that will assist you in gaining insight. You develop a great yearning to have an experience that is not contained within your body. You'll need affirmations and triggers if you're having problems making sense of your dreams due to out-of-body experiences.

Experiments in the Real World

Check to see whether you're having a dream at the moment. You have the ability to create a lucid dream from scratch in your subconscious. You are no longer in your physical body once you enter one of these dreams and become aware of it. The dream world vanishes at the end of the dream, leaving your body suspended in space. Put it into action every day and watch how your life changes. As a result, you will be able to recall details from your lucid dreams.

You should practice guided meditation every day.

These meditations are excellent since they help you relax and focus your mind when sleeping. These meditations can also be used to help you focus on a certain theme in your dreams.

While this may appear to be a simple task, there are numerous benefits to performing it on a regular basis. It assists you in becoming more aware of your dreams as well as relaxing and becoming more aware of your surroundings when you awaken.

Despite its apparent simplicity, performing it every day has a lot of advantages. This strategy enables you to remain alert and comfortable in your dreams while also being more aware of your surroundings. Examine your sleeping habits to evaluate if you're getting adequate rest. Examine your sleeping habits to evaluate if you're getting adequate rest. You'll need a lot of sleep to remember the dream clearly. This is useful for everyone, but it is especially important if you wish to have lucid dreams on a regular basis. Make certain that your sleep is restful and natural. If you can go asleep quickly and stay asleep for a lengthy period of time, your chances of having a lucid dream increase.

Guided Meditations for Lucid Dreaming

If you wish to utilize guided meditation to induce lucid dreams, here's a guide with some of the greatest meditations and instructions on how to apply them:

1. Progressive muscle relaxation. Each area of the body that you want to relax requires one minute of relaxation. This meditation can help you sleep more deeply and for a longer period of time each night. If you're having difficulties sleeping, try to give your body the rest it needs.
2. Breathing exercises are a type of relaxation. This is yet another wonderful, guided meditation that may help you sleep faster and relax your thoughts. Before attempting again, take a few more deep breaths in and out for another 20 seconds.
3. The third stage is to use affirmations. This is another guided meditation that can assist you in concentrating on a certain lucid dream. To accomplish the assignment, you must repeat a statement for ten minutes at night and recall a specific object or scene from your dreams. Here are some instances of statements:

When in doubt about whether you're dreaming or not, declaring "I'm dreaming" can be very helpful. Before inspecting your surroundings, you can ask yourself, "Am I dreaming?" and receive an answer before determining whether or not you are dreaming.

If you have problems having lucid dreams or have a lot of them, it's best to announce aloud, "Tonight, I'm going to dream lucidly." By repeating this comment ten minutes before bedtime, you can ensure a clear dream without expending much effort.

4. Fourth, a crystal ball of some kind. It's time for yet another incredible guided meditation to help you attain lucid dreaming! You can either listen to someone else say the words or utter them yourself. Despite being a little more challenging, this strategy has been demonstrated to be effective for a large number of people.

5. Binaural beats trump stereophonic beats. This is a supplement to help you have more vivid dreams. While this method is less technical than utilizing a crystal ball, it is more successful, especially if you are new to lucid dreaming.
6. Self-awareness is number six on the list. Meditating is a sort of meditation. This page also includes a lucid dreaming meditation guide. Because this is a genuine meditation, you will be able to maintain a state of tranquility and relaxation for the rest of your days. It's also relaxing to listen to before bed.
7. It is critical to remember that brainwave training is essential. This method of achieving lucid dreams can be achieved by listening to binaural beats designed specifically for this purpose or by utilizing an app such as Binaural Beats Meditation. A stereo headphone jack allows you to listen to the tone in the ear that best matches the beat frequency; you can even listen to the tone while wearing headphones. When your brain detects binaural beats, it forms an audio wave, which is then sent to your ears. Your brain creates this illusion by mixing those two tones with the ambient noise. As a result of this approach, an additional tone may be heard between these two original frequencies.
8. Agni Fire Therapy is an energy healing technique. This guided meditation is excellent for lucid dreaming! Even if you do not focus on a specific subject while sleeping, you will notice a significant shift in a short period of time - your dreams will become much more vivid and strong after twenty minutes of use once a day.
9. Brainwaves are generated (number nine). This is an online program that allows you to capture your brainwaves and utilize them as lucid dreaming music.
10. If you pay attention, you may be able to detect a subliminal message, which is an unconscious communication that your conscious mind can detect. This means you can hear it even

if you aren't aware of it, which is really beneficial for lucid dreaming.

Chapter 20:
Predicting Aura

What exactly is an aura, and how does it function? You've almost certainly heard the term before, but you might not know what it means unless you look it up. Every one of us has one. This is something that all living things do, but for the time being, we'll concentrate on humans. The energy environment that surrounds you gives you a sense of your own particular identity. Auras are a type of light or energy that emerges from another person without physical contact and can provide information about that person's characteristics. Aura reading is a difficult skill to learn and takes a lot of effort.

Auras are three-dimensional, oval, egg-shaped electromagnetic energy fields that have been observed throughout the history of the earth and humanity. Mystics and other clarividents have historically characterized this occurrence as waves and colored bands coming from the object of sight, among other things. The usage of halo images in religious iconography is another way to communicate this wonder.

The aura primarily reflects the individual's energy makeup, which carries information about their emotional, physical, cognitive, and spiritual well-being. This encompasses present as well as previous symptoms. A person's aura's size and color fluctuate on a regular basis in reaction to their current state and health, and the aura can also alter substantially over time.

People with a high level of charm have more clout in their professions and are more effective at persuading others. Confident and healthy people's auras remain longer and are more effective at blocking bad energy.

Individuals who are concerned about their own well-being and are enduring mental or physical challenges will have thinner auras and will seek to protect themselves from outside influences. While everyone's aura is unique, the ordinary person's aura is unstable, if not unhealthy, and it depicts everyone's constantly shifting moods and compulsive thinking.

When one engages in significant spiritual action, the aura becomes solid and unwavering, reflecting one's mental training. Increased consciousness results from an appreciation for the aura's value and the necessity of protecting oneself from negativity in the same way one protects oneself from illness and poor weather.

Expanding auras, in general, give a more expansive and pleasant sense of well-being. The word "energy retraction" refers to a decrease in the amount of available energy.

Even if it evolves, a healthy aura will retain its character and ability to maintain homeostasis in the face of changing external conditions. A person's aura fluctuates due to a multitude of factors, including their health, weather and other environmental stimuli, interpersonal relationships, cognitive patterns, emotions, and spiritual practice, to name a few.

Another critical factor to consider is the velocity of the planets. Celestial body configurations have an effect on everything, sometimes silently and sometimes not so quietly. Many signs prefer to display their auras in a unique fashion that reflects the underlying patterns of the sign, and the aura carries the individual's astrological plans.

When compared to their potential, the majority of auras are very calm, explosive, and mild in comparison to their entire size. Positive auras attract people, whilst negative auras repel them. This rule is known for deviating when manipulators use deception to make themselves appear desirable or when they work in low-incentive circumstances.

You can put on a strong mask that deceives others into believing in you unless they are more perceptive than you. Another alternative is to be overwhelmed by a beautiful aura because it broadens your horizons, or to be horrified by one because it reminds you of your own inadequacies.

Although auras are regarded to be extensions of individual souls, a process known as 'auric coupling' can temporarily or permanently combine two or more auras for a period of time. Maybe two friends had a long and thorough chat, or maybe two persons had recently engaged in physical proximity.

A person's aura might be a single color or a spectrum of colors that surrounds their body. Consider enlisting the assistance of a friend to practice observing someone's aura against a white background. If the background is too small, just her head and shoulders are okay; if the background is too small, only her head and shoulders are acceptable. This is the best approach for beginners to practice since the neutral background allows the colors in the surrounding region to stand out more. Other colors may distract them, so encourage them to dress in as neutral a manner as possible. Avoid places where you might get sidetracked or lose attention.

You can not only see someone's aura, but you can also feel it rather powerfully. That's a lot easier than detecting someone's aura because you've almost certainly sensed the aura of someone else before. You must first learn about auras and your own energetic presence. It's straightforward, and there are two approaches. Rub your palms together and then separate them till you reach the next level. Continue to draw them closer together, observing how your energy alters and grows as you get closer. Furthermore, the inverse is correct. Firmly press your palms together for 30 seconds to a minute, depending on your grip strength. Then, exactly as you did with the first treatment, carefully separate them and gradually recombine them. Take note of how the energy in your hands appeared to be closer together in both circumstances, despite the fact that they were not in contact at all?

A visual and energetic reading of the aura is required to perceive the person for whom you are reading, their personality, and their current emotional and mental state. When others approach you, you have the potential to absorb their worries and apprehensions, as well as their demeanor. With this information, you may personalize the reading to the topic at hand. As a psychic, you'll quickly realize that no two people are the same, and hence no two readings are the same. Based on your premonition insights, you may want to explain premonitions to others using a variety of ways, techniques, and strategies.

Your aura is an energy sphere that surrounds you. He or she is a mirror image of yourself and your current state of being. It's possible that negative energy has burdened and impeded it; as a result, it has to be cleansed and revitalized.

Furthermore, if you are experiencing a period of stagnation in your life, your aura may be sluggish. Take some time to consider and examine the problem to see if you can identify the cause of the problem. If you believe they apply to you in the way you believe they do, you must address them, no matter how tough. If you maintain that level of strength, it will have an effect on your psychological abilities, making you feel too lethargic or powerful to develop your gift correctly. Treat your aura's problems like you would a disease or a broken bone.

Individuals who lack the necessary grounding and stability to deal with the opportunities that psychic abilities provide can develop psychic abilities. Instead of being a blessing, information confuses and perplexes life; having too much information is not a desired thing.

Another type of psychological abuse is the purposeful cultivation of insight for egoistic or damaging purposes. Psychic abuse has a lengthy and well-documented history. Psychic talents aren't frequently associated with spiritual growth. Many psychics with great talents are neither intelligent nor evolved, and vice versa. Maintain a high level of self-awareness and exercise caution when disclosing or expressing your thoughts to others.

As the ego matures and the universe is discovered as a result of spiritual practice and advancement, psychic ability emerges organically. The occurrence is most likely magical or horrific (or both), and if it troubles you, you'll want to figure out how to deal with it while keeping your skill under control. More information about a subject can be quite useful, and sometimes all you need is confirmation that you are not mad.

As a result of this training, the ability to perceive or feel the energy in a person, place, or item improved. Other people's energy is normally required for you to understand it, and the other person has the right to refuse you access if they so desire.

In these situations, you are frequently unable to perceive what you desire, and you are unable to act on your desire without permission. The only exceptions are when you're attempting to learn something new or, in more severe cases, when you're insulting the other person's goals and attempting to suffocate them with your energy. To begin, pay attention to the energy that surrounds us:

- Making your workplace a pleasant place to work is a wonderful place to start. For example, a park, zoo, restaurant, or a member of your family.
- Sit in your favorite spot and notice how you're feeling.
- Experiment with perceiving beyond your five senses and cultivate an awareness of the energy in your surroundings. Maybe you'd like to close your eyes for a bit.
- Take a walk about the neighborhood to check for changes in energy levels—one site may be more positive or intense than others.
- As you exit your shelter, notice how the energy fluctuates in response to the surroundings. What do you believe you're seeing? What do you believe you're seeing?

Auras Seen in a New Light

Seeing energy is a more refined and elevated way of expressing it. Many individuals have seen it, only to dismiss it as a fabrication of their imagination. Light, color, or a moving field may be discernible around a person's body contour.

When you first begin to detect auras, you will observe what looks to be a neck and waves in the sky. It will take a long time and a lot of experience to master colors and other design components. Those born with a natural propensity for it learned how to do it in previous incarnations.

There are undoubtedly more people who can see auras than we believe. People typically keep such information hidden for fear of being called "strange" or "unstable," as well as rejected or rebuked by their peers. Those that have this capacity, on the other hand, may choose to use it very well on occasion. A variety of strategies are available for training the eyes to record faint information in order to discern auras:

- Enter a plant room and turn off all the lights. A strong, bright, and neutral wall works nicely as a backdrop for the plant's foliage.
- Instead of looking at the plant directly in the eyes, take a look at it with your peripheral vision. After several repetitions, a fuzzy shape forms around the plant.
- Following that, you'll be able to interact with both animals and humans.

Chapter 21:
Dream Interpretation

Empaths regularly study dreams to discover if they are related to reality. This demonstrates the ability to travel beyond realms and engage with energy outside the boundaries of conventional knowledge.

Empaths frequently have free-fall dreams. These dreams are associated with the advent of spiritual energies. They're also interpretive, with many people believing they represent the necessity to find the strength to face difficulties in daily life. Sequential dreams, which can be quite structured, can relate to dream events. This keeps track of events so you can comprehend what happened in real life.

Creativity-related dreams can be motivating. Empaths can gather ideas from their dreams by watching and interacting with them. Dreamscapes can be bright and colorful as a result of empaths' creative imaginations and extensive experience connecting with diverse energy sources. Empaths may experience very unpleasant and frightening nightmares. Because of their extraordinary sensitivity, even minor information can become engraved in their minds until it can be resolved. You might wish to attempt some sleep meditation and energy clearing practices before bed to help in the production of pleasant dreams.

Empaths must be prepared to cope with the emotional toll that vivid dreams can impose. Many of them will be able to fully explain and interpret their dreams as long as they match their subconscious and spiritual truths. Even if you're not aware that you're an Empath, it's easy to live your life as an energetic sponge. Those who are unaware of their skills will absorb these feelings and energy wherever they go, oblivious to the reason for their presence. Regardless of whether the feeling is caused, it may manifest as an unexpected ailment, as well as overwhelming anxiety or grief.

To maintain control of your empathy and avoid overload, you'll need to practice self-care and safety practices. The consciousness of one's physical state of being is becoming increasingly significant. As an empath, you may experience neurological system overheating and must recognize the symptoms and take corrective action. Breathing strategies to help you recover your center of gravity and drop your heart rate It's critical to be aware of your emotions after spending time with someone. It will not take you long to recognize the persons and situations that could jeopardize your health and safety.

One type of self-care is interacting with and activating your chakras. If you're familiar with the seven Chakras, you'll understand how they can assist you in controlling your body's energy and emotions. It is feasible to eliminate all stored energy and strengthen all of the body's energy centers by draining all stored energy and strengthening all of the body's energy centers for only a few minutes each day. Concentrating on a chakra while meditating and performing breathing exercises is a simple approach to demonstrate how you can send pure, clean energy into the area while eliminating any negative energies, as shown in the diagram. Many aspects of yoga are dedicated to balancing and harmonizing chakras, which can be incredibly good for empaths who are feeling overburdened.

The majority of us have fantasized about falling from enormous heights at some point in our lives. It's a very common and frightening dream, and some people believe that if you wake up from it, you'll die. This is obviously false, with no truth to it! So, what does this all mean? What does this mean exactly?

According to dream analysts, this dream is related to personal concerns in the dreamer's life. You claim it's an indication of an out-of-control situation, and I agree. As a result, you may find that at critical junctures in your life, you must shift your course of action or choose an alternate path. It could also imply that you are fearful and concerned about a certain situation in your life, such as your career or a personal relationship.

Lately, everything has felt like a dream. Have you ever fantasized about passing up an opportunity because you were late for a meeting? This type of dream might be confusing and unpleasant. This is a reflection of the concerns you are now experiencing in your life. You may be apprehensive about impending changes or your ability to fulfill present projects. If you purposefully arrive late for appointments or dates, you're definitely overworked and don't have enough time to get there. If you arrive late at the airport and miss your flight, it indicates that you don't have enough time to complete the task at hand. Accepting sufficiently tough work is the most effective treatment.

It might be quite frustrating to have a dream about hunting for a toilet when we are in desperate need of one. In this case, you may discover that whatever you're starring at while attempting to relieve yourself is actually a toilet. Despite the embarrassment, the impulse to choose a location is motivated by nature. According to dream specialists, this could be a depiction of our daily anxieties and fears. This demonstrates that we have become so preoccupied with serving the needs of others that we have forgotten about our own. It could also mean that we struggle to express ourselves in everyday situations.

Snakes appear in your dreams.

A dream in which you see or are bitten by food can be rather unsettling. On the other hand, the vast majority of dream specialists say that the dream depicts temptations, danger, and forbidden sexuality. Snakes represent transformation and healing, but they can also act as a warning sign that something horrible is about to happen. Snakes chasing you indicate that you are evading a critical requirement.

If a snake chases after you, this indicates that something in your life has gotten out of hand, whether it's your health or a relationship. If you have a dream about fighting a snake, it indicates that you are going through some changes or challenges in your life. If you are compelled to do something you dislike or if something unexpected happens, you may be unsatisfied. If you get bitten by a snake in your dream, it suggests you are confronted with risky situations that could devastate your life, and you must act swiftly.

This is a prevalent aspiration among folks who have completed high school and are now working in a performance-related sector. It's linked to self-criticism and a desire to live a longer life. This dream, according to dream interpreters, signifies a dread of failure and anxiety. It might also represent the beginning of a new phase in your life or a future event that will require you to make a decision. It could also mean that you have poor self-esteem or confidence and are concerned that your current path is not the best one for you.

Dreams about pregnancy

This is again another dream that can be interpreted in numerous ways. It heralds the start of a new chapter as well as a new task. According to dream analyst Loewenberg, this is a nice dream that indicates a woman's capacity for growth and development will continue to improve. This also signals the start of a new thinking, direction, or undertaking. It could also be the result of a woman's anxiety of becoming incompetent as a mother at some time during her parenting career. This dream foretells increased monetary fortune, the budding of romantic feelings, and a drastic change.

Flight dreams

If you are afraid of heights, flying dreams can be both horrifying and fascinating. Some dream interpreters feel it denotes liberty and independence and that it may represent a previous attempt to flee in your life.

Other dream experts feel that if you can't fly in your dream, you're either attempting to attain your life goals or something is impeding your success. They claim that flying solo represents freedom and liberation from social limitations or that you are liberated from whatever has been suffocating you.

Dreaming about your partner being unfaithful

This dream may be exceedingly unpleasant, forcing someone to ask aloud after having it, "What if it's true?" According to dream psychologists, such nightmares do not signify that your sweetheart is unfaithful to you or that you are unfaithful to your sweetheart. It could be an indication that you're terrified of being unfaithful or that you've been tricked in the past and don't want to be duped again.

You have the potential to stretch the boundaries of reality! Such nightmares may also signify a breakdown in communication and a lack of trust in your relationship. You may also have dreams about not spending enough time with your lover due to work demands or physical distance.

Dreams about tooth loss

This dream might be interpreted in a number of different ways. Some dream analysts believe that teeth signify power and trust and that the dreamer's loss of trust, as well as his or her ability to become aggressive and resolute, could be an indication of something happening in the dreamer's personal life. It can indicate a breakdown in some cases, pregnancy in others, and sexual arousal in still others. According to some dream interpreters, this dream could also represent insecurity over one's own attractiveness and appearance. It may also be nervous about speaking or fearful of saying anything embarrassing.

Desires to be seen by the public

It might be really frustrating to have a dream in which you are naked at work or school! Such a scene, according to dream specialists, depicts feelings of vulnerability, insecurity, embarrassment, and humiliation in one's life. This is a regular occurrence for folks who have discovered a new career route that requires them to interact with members of the general population.

Death is a reoccurring theme in a number of my nightmares.

Almost everyone awakens in pain from their nightmares. Dreams concerning a departed family member or acquaintance are possible. Some people feel that keeping your dreams to yourself can aid in their realization! This, however, is not the case. This dream, according to dream interpreters, signifies shifting anxiety.

This can occur if you are terrified of change since you don't know what will happen throughout your organization. Only the cries of time's unrelenting march can be heard. This dream may also imply that the dreamer intends to end their life by inflicting pain on others. This could be because of a challenging task, a relationship, or a painful event in their history. Some experts say this isn't a pipe dream but rather a desire to explore new research possibilities.

Chapter 22:
The Chakras

The chakra most closely resembles the spiritual realm's condition of balance and eternal order.

When a chakra is balanced and healthy, it may emit the appropriate amount of pleasant energy. While the energy is flowing freely, it does not hinder or control other portions of your body.

In this condition, the functioning of the chakras is readily seen. When your chakras are functional and balanced, you can emit positive energy and have wonderful colored auras. Your spirits have been elevated, and you are always in a good mood. The better your physical health will be, the more balanced and vigilant your chakras are.

Chakras that are out of balance are equivalent to hormones that are out of balance. If you learn how to work with your chakra points and other psychological self-healing methods, your emotional state will drastically improve. Instead, you can guard yourself against negative energy and mental baggage that seeks to bring you down rapidly.

From your sacrum, the triangle bone at the base of your spine, to the summit of your skull, in ascending sequence because each chakra corresponds to a certain area of the body, various colors, natural products, and physical routines can be employed to soothe and treat each chakra.

As previously said, each chakra connects to a different part of the physical body or an emotion that may be felt in that area of the body. When your chakras are out of balance, your body's wisdom manifests as symptoms such as pain, sickness, or emotional compulsion. If these signs are ignored, long-term problems may occur. Infantile traumas, as well as new injuries, infections, or discomfort, may have long-term bodily consequences.

Meditation, yoga, lifestyle modifications, crystal treatment, essential oils, and Reiki are all methods for balancing your chakras. Using these techniques, you may help nurture a specific chakra, which is beneficial if you have discovered a blockage in that area, or you can develop an overall chakra balance practice that targets the entire system, among other things.

Remember that chakra imbalances and blockages can show in a variety of ways, making it difficult to pinpoint which chakra is out of balance and producing problems. If you're having difficulties with your body, it's ideal to begin with dietary changes and then incorporate bodywork such as Reiki, yoga, massage, or acupuncture into your regimen. If your concerns are primarily mental or emotional in nature, begin by using crystals or essential oils, meditating, writing, and scheduling time to unwind.

If one or more of our chakras are blocked, energy cannot flow freely through us. When a chakra in our body is obstructed, a segment of our life is usually affected. This is why clearing and balancing your chakras is so crucial. It's important to remember that your chakras are interconnected and flow via one another; as a result, even if one of your chakras is blocked, you'll lose your equilibrium and become influenced by the chakras.

Chakra system balance has a variety of benefits, including making you feel happier, healthier, and more connected to yourself and the rest of the world. Each chakra is hampered by a specific challenge, and when balanced, each chakra contributes to your life in some way. In this section, I'll go through the overall benefits of having all seven chakras balanced.

Balanced chakras provide the following benefits:

- Your chakras are opened, allowing physical and emotional energy to flow freely. If you are still coping with unresolved grief or vulnerability, you may be experiencing blocked emotional energy. Once this energy has been released, you will feel more joy, vitality, and less vulnerability.

- Cleaning the chakras increases drive and self-confidence. You'll have a better probability of success in all of your undertakings and will be more likely to meet your goals.
- You will look and feel younger, and you will be healthier than you have ever been with unobstructed chakras.
- You will discover that your intuition becomes more sensitive to your needs. Blockages in the chakras may cause you to distrust others and feel unable to think or feel. When your chakras are in good condition, you can have more faith in your intuition and have fewer reservations about it.
- You'll be able to create deeper emotional connections with others. When your chakras are in harmony, you may be able to connect with your emotions more profoundly, resulting in deeper emotional experiences. Even though you are more aware of your emotions, you have complete control over them, ensuring that they do not overwhelm you. A balanced chakra system is the first step in efficiently managing one's emotional state and connecting with the emotions of others in interpersonal relationships.
- We are all participants in the fight against dishonesty in some way. Whether it's to avoid shame or to keep others safe. If your chakras are balanced, you will be able to appreciate the significance of the truth and communicate it more effectively. Even if the cold, hard reality is tough to accept, hearing the truth from others will help you grow in wisdom.
- You'll become more at ease and confident in your own skin as you practice. It's no secret that we all have times when we feel self-conscious about our appearance. When your chakra system is functioning properly, you may feel more confident and at peace with yourself, including your sexuality.
- Chakra balance might help you link your thoughts. Many common ailments, such as stress, worry, insomnia, melancholy, and dependency, can be eased by balancing your chakras. A chakra system that is well-balanced corresponds to a life that is well-balanced. When your chakra system is in good health, you

may be able to think more clearly and experience a rise in creativity.
- Your mental toughness will develop as a result. This implies you'll be able to take more abuse and, as a result, kill the rest of the planet. The world can be cruel at times, and we can sustain physical and emotional suffering as a result of a variety of conditions. With a healthy chakra system, you'll be able to handle better with life's harsh realities, and you'll be able to reject or ignore them depending on the scenario.
- When your chakras are balanced, your overall health improves, and your immune system becomes more capable of resisting disease. If your body is chaotic and out of balance, you will be more vulnerable to illness. You'll be happy and healthy for the rest of your life if you keep your chakras and body in harmony.

These are little benefits of a balanced chakra system, but they have the potential to transform you into someone quite different. Many of the activities we do now were never meant to be done in the past. We shouldn't be worried about a hundred different things at once. A vast percentage of people are affected by out-of-balance chakras.

Many modern-day components have the ability to clog and destabilize our chakras, causing them to become imbalanced or clogged. The modern world is designed to annoy us. To begin fighting back, we could focus on chakra alignment. After you have balanced your chakras, you will be more prepared to deal with life's challenges that sometimes throw us off balance.

Chakras, which are located in the spiritual or energy body, are equivalent to key organs in the physical body. It is critical to keep your chakras in good health since misaligned chakras can lead to physical illness. According to one study, physical ailments develop first, followed by energy or spiritual ailments. The chakras also signify energy entry and departure points into and out of the body. To awaken the Kundalini, your chakras must be robust and healthy.

Because the spirit and physical bodies are inextricably linked, it is critical to keep your chakras clean and functioning properly. The chakras, especially the major chakras of the body, allow energy to freely move throughout the body. If a person is ill, one or more of their chakras is most certainly malfunctioning.

It's important to note that the chakras affect both your emotional and spiritual well-being as well as your physical health. A strong root chakra, for example, indicates that you are in control of your life. If your heart chakra is in good health, you may expect your life to be filled with harmony and love. As you can see, the state and health of your chakras have a significant impact on your overall quality of life.

Chakras are mystical energy vortexes that manifest as circular expressions of vitality when they vibrate at a precise rate.

Although everyone possesses several chakras, only a few of them are used in tantric and yogic ceremonies. These chakras represent the full range of human activity, from the most annoying to the most serene.

Chakras are physiological and clairvoyant foci with structures that correspond to classical descriptions of energy centers. These functional hubs are found at the junctions of spinal segments rather than within the spinal cord itself. When the spinal line is split crosswise at various levels, the faint problem resembles a lotus flower, and the ascending and descending nerve pathways resemble the *nadis*. Many publications and articles say that the chakras are energy storage centers, but this is not true.

A chakra, similar to a power shaft, increases the transmission of electrical wires throughout the neighborhood to better sites, houses, and streetlights. The nadis that arise from each chakra carry prana between the two coverings. The nadis have a forward and backward pranic movement that is roughly equal to the flow progression of replacement electrical wiring. The nadis that connect the chakra to the ongoing correspondence and the expected response enter and exit the chakra.

The development of the chakras might also contribute to an increase in psychic capacity. As a result, you'll spend a lot of time during your training dealing with your chakras. The body is comprised of seven primary chakras that must be comprehended.

The Root Chakra

The first out of seven chakras that exist is the root chakra. It is found at the base of the spinal cord in the human body. The color red represents the root chakra. To represent this chakra, visualize a red spinning wheel, a red circle, or a red flower arrangement.

Because it is located at the base of the other three chakras, it serves as the basis for all living things. The primary objectives are to provide a solid foundation and sustain stability.

A strong root chakra provides a solid foundation and a sense of stability. It is also related to physical security and identification. If you wish to feel more grounded, devote some attention to your root chakra.

If you are feeling wobbly or confused, you may be suffering from a weak root chakra. Greed, avarice, and even eating disorders are symptoms of a damaged root chakra.

It's also crucial to remember that the kundalini is located in the root chakra; thus, focusing on your kundalini while also focusing on your root chakra is natural.

This chakra, often known as the sex chakra, is orange in hue. It is associated with the chakras of sensuality and emotion. This chakra governs emotions, feelings, relationships, physiological pleasures, and preferences. Some say it's three centimeters below the navel, while others say it's right in the vaginal area.

A healthy holy chakra indicates that you are content with your current connections and have no difficulty expressing your emotions. It also suggests the possibility of sensory-based life perception. It corresponds to the well-being chakra.

Unhappy relationships and trouble expressing your excitement may indicate a weakened holy chakra. Allowing your emotions to run wild increases the likelihood that they will rule and manage your feelings, particularly your sensual ones, rather than the other way around.

Yellow is the most popular color. Yellow. The chakra is in charge of an individual's willpower. It is linked to autonomy, self-esteem, self-worth, and the ability to trust. If you wish to recognize your own inner strength, you should concentrate your efforts on this chakra.

Low self-esteem and respect indicate a weakened solar plexus chakra. You should also be cautious not to activate it too frequently or too frequently. A lack of humility can manifest itself in a variety of ways, including being too boastful or unattractive.

The Heart Chakra can be found in the center of the chest.

It has a greenish tint to it. It is the epicenter of universal affection and pity. This is a discussion concerning your emotions and relationships with other sentient beings. All spiritual gurus, including the Buddha and Jesus, had completely developed heart chakras, which resulted in compassion and love for everyone they came into contact with. If you wish to increase your compassion capacity, you should work on growing your heart chakra. To create a powerful heart chakra, the Kundalini must first be aroused.

Egotism and contempt for other sentient beings could be symptoms of an underdeveloped heart chakra. On the other hand, an overdeveloped heart chakra may lead to you being abused by others. Unfortunately, some individuals mistake kindness for weakness.

The Throat Chakra is located in the center of the throat.

The blue-hued neck chakra is housed in the throat. It governs how people communicate and how they utilize words. You will be able to express yourself more freely and connect with your creative side if your throat chakra is appropriately developed. If, on the other hand, you struggle to talk or write, you should work on your throat chakra. Every member recognizes the importance of communication in any relationship.

Ajna Chakra

The next chakra in the sequence is the Ajna chakra, which has a blue tone. The location of the Ajna chakra between the brows is well recognized. As a result, if you want to develop strong intuition and psychic vision, you should concentrate on this chakra.

The Ajna chakra is essential for the development of clairvoyance since it is the seat of intuition. Vision is defined as unobstructed vision. It has the ability to see beyond the range of human vision. When you visualize something, for example, you may assume you're employing the power of the Ajna chakra to regulate your prana.

It's always the finest way to boost the functioning of your Ajna chakra and other chakras. This chakra can be stimulated by any sort of meditation that includes imagery. This chakra is also referred to as the "bridge" between this world and the next, in the same way as the Ajna chakra is referred to as the "bridge" between this world and the crown chakra; which is referred to as the "hub of universal knowledge."

The Crown Chakra

The seventh chakra, which is violet in color, is the head and neck chakra. To reach illumination, you must invest time and effort in the growth of your third eye chakra. The chakra that must be cultivated in order to acquire this state of awareness is the Buddha mind, also known as Christ consciousness. This chakra is the key to understanding how life and spirituality are intertwined.

It's vital to recognize that the chakras' functions are inextricably linked. Another example is that in order to have a healthy relationship with others, you must work on your throat chakra, heart chakra, and even sacred chakra. As a result, when exercising, you must be careful not to disregard any of these chakras. Indeed, in order to really awaken Kundalini, all seven chakras must be in good operating order.

Chapter 23:
Grounding

We shall initially construct our physical bodies and 3D environments for a variety of reasons before engaging in any higher-dimensional activity. Here are a couple of instances:

1. To avoid being badly impacted by a large amount of intense cosmic energy
2. In order to avoid future grief, it is necessary to look for oneself.
3. To safeguard our personal safety.
4. Increasing our awareness of the energy flow throughout our entire body.
5. To have our efforts recognized and backed up by others.

If you're already a psychic or are familiar with comparable concepts, you'll understand exactly what I mean when I say this list, and you may opt to continue with guided meditation after that. Some of you may have desired a relaxing pre-performance ritual that would allow you to give your all in a divine setting while remaining grounded, secure, and protected by your spirit guides and instructors.

Those of us who embark on this spiritual journey are looking for something more than ourselves, something that will give our life meaning and fulfillment. We may have held recollections of previous lifetimes as spiritual thinkers and seekers, and this yearning may have been etched on our souls for generations. The job of seeker or seer may be genetically encoded in our souls. It's very likely that we'll return to it after each incarnation on Earth, awakening with a burning desire to remember our divine origins and communicate with others about how wonderful this spiritual existence is, with all of its discoveries, possibilities, and delights, as well as our divine origins.

Many of us will experience spiritual awakenings or rediscover spirituality as a result of tragedy or loss, or years of suffering and effort, to name a few instances. We could be looking for answers or attempting to recuperate from a traumatic event in our life. Unhealed causes and soul contracts can play a variety of roles in spiritual awakening, and we may approach spiritual activities with an unconscious desire to avoid the most unpleasant aspects of our lives that result from these unhealed elements of our awareness. As we spiritually evolve, we will unavoidably recognize that it is a tremendous opportunity to enrich, grow, and transform our physical earthly realities into something even more extraordinary.

Grounding is especially necessary if you've been through trauma, abuse, or some form of emotional turmoil that has caused you to want to abandon your body. As previously stated, your spiritual practice should eventually serve as a vehicle for heart and mind healing, allowing you to re-appreciate and love your existence. If your illness appears to be out of control or unpredictable, you must seek professional assistance. Qualified specialists can help you process your feelings and provide a safe place for you to cry and recover in a respectful environment.

It's impossible for me to picture a single student who hasn't suffered sadness or heartbreak during our initial sessions together as a spiritual teacher, guide, counselor, and coach with extraordinary sensitivity. Individuals with strong sensitivity may find the human problem itself disturbing. We are at risk of being misunderstood, injured, or abandoned from the moment we are conceived. It is critical to identify the myriad ways in which life can injure, shock, or deceive us in order to focus as much as possible on our own rehabilitation, to behave responsibly, with clarity of mind, and with a clean conscience for the ultimate well-being of all, including ourselves. Accepting, appreciating, and paying attention to what the human condition and life itself have to give is the first step in this crucial healing process.

After experiencing trauma, many of us seek spiritual or healing disciplines that are unrelated to, or at least hardly addressed in many respects in relation to, our daily lives before going on our own personal recovery journeys. We may be fearful because we are unable to properly engage with our bodies. Even if we have no notion where we are, we may feel separated from our human bodily experience and a strong yearning to return home.

In my professional life, I saw numerous kids who had this wound — pupils who continually stumbled over their belongings had mishaps and found it nearly impossible to concentrate. Because these sensations are generally indicative of trauma, anxiety, and suicide attempts, grounding oneself may be the first step toward countering these trends. If you identify with any of the above, it is vital that you spend as much time as possible practicing grounding meditation before proceeding to the next phase.

It's possible that you'll require many months of orientation before you're ready to begin the program, which is pretty common. If you're not used to being grounded, you may grow tired of it as you practice. This is merely a sign that your body is adjusting to its own weight as well as the general heaviness of your Earth experience, which you may have chosen to disregard. Nonetheless, you can be certain that you will quickly come to love the third dimension and all that it has to offer. Throughout the day, you'll be introduced to the fascinating variations and diversity that 5D travelers provide, as well as learning how to navigate across many dimensions.

Cosmic Energies with Force in Contact

For the second reason, it is necessary to ground yourself before engaging in any mental activity. This will prepare you for the tremendous amount of mental energy that will be poured over you in order to awaken your heart and mind to a higher level of consciousness.

As science is currently showing us, everything in the cosmos is made up of frequencies. Every item, living or inanimate, visible, or invisible, as well as each of us, has a frequency. Even the ground vibrates at a specific frequency, and as sensitive beings, we are continually exposed to and recognize a wide range of frequencies. When we come into prolonged contact with specific energies or emotions, our entire field of energy is impacted, and our brains notice a shift in frequency even when we are not dealing with these possibilities.

Based on their studies of these frequencies and vibratory fields, scientists observed that certain items or groups vibrate or oscillate at a very rapid rate, i.e., at higher frequencies, whilst others vibrate or oscillate at a slower or slower rate.

When we open up to the entire cosmos of possible frequencies in certain areas of spiritual and psychic development, we can come into contact with frequencies that vibrate faster and are much greater than those with which we have a connection in three-dimensional awareness, and it is critical that we are able to deal with a dramatic change in the frequencies in these situations.

If we are not completely grounded, these frequencies - the vibrations of angels, spiritual guides, and other celestial messengers – may surprise us as they interact with our energy field.

A sudden influx of heavenly energies, particularly those of the most ardent Spiritual seekers, can be overwhelming and even dangerous in the hands of an untrained practitioner, mentalist, or healer.

In the event of abrupt and rapid spiritual awakenings, we don't always have time to develop ground before high frequencies make contact with us, so we have to go with the flow and learn on our own, via trial and error, until the high frequencies make contact with us. While grounding is required before dealing with these higher energies, our strong and conscious connection to Mother Earth will physically pull us into the 3D currents, keeping us connected to a safer and more stable frequency. She can not only survive but also appreciate these higher frequencies as a result of her rigorous training and deep appreciation for the procedures required to become a healthy and efficient Fifth Dimension Practitioner.

If you're not sure what I mean, simply know that connecting with higher frequencies is usually a lovely experience that should leave you feeling uplifted, reassured, valued, and totally confident in your own skin. If you feel confused, baffled, frustrated, terrified, or freaked out at any point in this book, you are almost certainly not operating at higher frequencies and should look into some of the energy clarity ideas further.

Finally, these energies should never be feared; their transcendental beauty is genuinely stunning, putting a firm grip on our terrestrial reality all the more important in this scenario. These energies have the ability to produce such amazing experiences in the heart, body, and mind that they may result in physical disappointment and disillusionment. When survivors of near-death experiences return to their normal lives, they frequently express extreme sadness and alienation from all that was truly precious, gorgeous, and spectacular in their past existence. Pursuing happiness, maintaining a feeling of self-awareness, and engaging in daily contact with nature can all help to alleviate unpleasant moods.

ùThese higher frequencies can induce physiological symptoms in some circumstances, as well as being unpleasant and mentally distressing if we are not accustomed to them. Mild headaches, dizziness, and even weird plexus cramping are all possible side effects. We are significantly less likely to encounter symptoms if we can develop a sense of how energy circulates throughout the system; nevertheless, if we do, we will be much more able to recognize and address them swiftly and efficiently. Grounding strategies are vital for self-care in the realm of new energy work.

We are at ease in our surroundings, secure in our physical condition and confident in our talents. We are connected to our bodily selves when we feel grounded. When we are unsure of ourselves, separated from our bodies, or contemplating escape and dissociation from physical reality, we become more sensitive to foreign energies moving through our energy environment. Consider the case of a tree with a high number of roots. They remain firm even in the face of the strongest gusts, even during a storm, and confront the issue head-on. When the roots of a tree are weak or underdeveloped, it can easily topple over, even in a light breeze.

Deep-rooted trees may be able to get more water and nutrients from the soil, helping them to grow stronger. By whatever means, the intruders are not easily intimidated or threatened.

Before you can begin your spiritual practice, you must first understand a few basic energy skills. These exercises will help you learn how energy interacts and moves between the mind, body, and spirit, and thus how to engage in spiritual activity. This enables you to help others by working with high-frequency energies and detecting bad energy more rapidly. These negative emotions aren't necessarily the result of something "out there" attempting to hurt us.

They can be a precursor to our own inner resistance or shadow work, both of which must be addressed at some point in order to achieve the highest levels of spiritual power. As a result of this voyage into the clear spiritual canal to which we have always been destined, our life will benefit from higher and better vibrational feelings, faster expressions, and improved feelings of serenity and well-being.

Grounding practices and guided grounding meditation, in general, will improve your ability to perceive and feel psychic energy as it moves through you.

As you may be aware or have learned in preparation for becoming a spiritual counselor, it is critical for us to maintain our own personal inner development and self-healing in our professional lives. While practically everyone may learn psychological skills, their own perspectives, injuries, prejudices, and world views all have an impact on the gifts they can offer. We can only connect with and aid the loving vibrations of the sky and earth on our own journeys if we are firmly rooted and allow a massive current of healing energy to flow consistently through the body.

As proven during ground meditation, grounding and connecting with appropriate energies may be quite pleasant and reassuring in practice.

As a result of this practice, we are able to connect with and draw from everything positive and useful in the universe.

If you consistently apply these tactics to your life, you will enhance your understanding and experience of never being alone in this world but rather of feeling loved and supported by an all-benevolent and loving universe.

Before embarking on any spiritual pursuit, we must constantly picture or conjure a form of protection. When we open our energy centers to pursue any form of spiritual endeavor, we open ourselves up to all kinds of invasions and disturbances. I'm not trying to scare you, and if you're sincerely interested in learning why mental defense and energy protection are so vital, you should conduct your own research. If you are an empath, you will not require my or anybody else's assistance in communicating your feelings. Empathy, in general, is unduly preoccupied with what might happen in the realm of energy exchange and connectedness.

A variety of energies should be avoided and kept away from the realms of mental, channeling, and healing. Allowing them access to your energy field by leaving it open is spiritually akin to leaving all of your doors and windows open while you're gone for the day. It is also known as going outside in the midst of winter without a coat, hat, gloves, or even shoes and expecting to get away with it.

If you are not an empath and are new to psychological work, you may be inclined to skip this part. Many of us have learned the value of protection as a result of repeated horrific experiences and spectacular awakenings, while others are convinced that these heinous acts are an essential part of their spiritual journey. However, I strongly advise you to avoid them if at all feasible. Take a lesson from these mistakes and use this thorough preparation strategy to ensure you don't repeat them.

Establishment Of Connection

You can now connect to the most powerful and loving energy in the universe and summon the assistance of your guides and superior teachers. This is when the real fun begins. If you're not sure what it means or why it's important, here's how I'd explain this phase in the process if you're not sure what it means or why it's important.

Individuals have a vast range of personalities, goals, ethics, and vibratory frequencies. When it comes to energy, the spectrum of frequencies in unseen worlds is similarly large. It would be naive to pretend otherwise, and if you find yourself drifting from an ungrounded to a grounded state of naiveté, now is a good time to halt, contemplate, breathe, regroup, and ensure that you conduct grounding meditations for several months before moving on to the next chapters of the book.

It is critical that we create a sacred setting before we begin our activity. Crystals, wisdom and wisdom, spiritual music, and singing are only a few of the accessible options. These are all extremely powerful weapons on their own, but when combined, two behaviors develop that, regardless of where we are or what instruments we use, establish an immutable sacred space: To begin, we must connect with our hearts and communicate our desire to help others on their spiritual journeys. The second point to make is that we are currently surrounded by some of the world's smartest and most caring mentors and teachers. It is likely that our guardian angels and guides, as well as archangels and ascenders, have opted to assist us at this time.

Avoid ego traps such as spiritual pride or hierarchical structures that may draw unwelcome attention to yourself. Maintain the mindset of a humble scholar who is always willing to learn, who trusts their intuition, and who is not deceived by the ringing of better or lower instruction. Allow your emotions to guide you, and let your inner radar of what feels good, light, cheerful, intelligent, and loving serve as your sole compass, guiding you to the person you'll become.

If you truly choose to serve and connect with divine love and light, you will have a deeper knowledge of the world and attract energies of the same frequency.

Mediums and channels communicate with deceased celebrities and great leaders via spiritual channels, yet they did not seek out these people on their spiritual journey. After all, recognized individuals on Earth are still humans, and if they were truly engaged, worried, and vocal while on the planet, they would seek means to ensure their everyday function.

Their light will be powerful as a result of a lifetime of spiritual service (or, indeed, numerous lives), and they will be exceptionally skilled at projecting their energy, love, and light through a medium or a channel. They will come to meet you if they believe you are willing to collaborate with them, in my experience. Even if it isn't part of your spiritual destiny, it's a beautiful ending if you can uplift people and help them improve their lives with the assistance of a departed man named John!

In addition to connecting with your heart and raising your vibration, the connecting process allows you to harmonize with and with your spiritual guides and teachers. Consider this portion of the process to be a new stage in the construction of your sensory energy, and if any of the energies provided to you as guides make you feel uncomfortable, call on God and your true guardian angels, pray, and reconnect with your higher self.

Chapter 24:
Connecting with Your Spirit Guides

Before you begin working with spirit guide meditation, make sure you're comfortable with the grounding, protection, and psychological connection techniques that will be used.

To create a spiritual connection with the Spirit, we must first understand how they communicate and how we might build our bonds with them through time.

Recognizing that our spiritual companions do not always communicate verbally is the first step toward comprehending them. Pictures, symbols, visual metaphors, and psychic downloads, which appear to be small packets of knowledge and comprehension, are common methods of communication.

Communication becomes easier as our degree of comfort with them rises, our ability to align our frequency with theirs improves, and they have a greater selection of communication styles and strategies to pick from.

Your developmental stage or the task's specific purpose may influence the kinds of communication you use. In some situations, such as when providing mediumship and your primary purpose is to demonstrate that there is life after death, you may receive an infinite number of images that are only relevant to the person hearing the message. When channeling a book, though, you may receive small packets of wisdom that explode into the pages as a flurry of words, information, and knowledge. When receiving text messages through mediumship, the capacity to hear or feel each word you're about to write a few seconds before you write it may be necessary.

Despite the fact that many individuals are captivated by the idea of a channel emerging from their bodies and allowing another entity to entirely occupy their conscience, channeling can be a deception. While this is an uncommon event, I consider a number of less dramatic media to be channeling since they allow for the reception of words, ideas, and concepts from a more spiritual being that is then conveyed through its consciousness to a more materialized sitter or audience.

In mediumship, on the other hand, the medium acts as a conduit between the general public and loved ones from the spiritual world, allowing messages to be heard, acknowledged, and understood by the general public before being passed on to the general public or the sitter.

As with so much in this profession, the two identities will inevitably become confused and distorted. In some cases, media can devolve into inspired, seemingly channeled speeches, and channels may appear to listen to and receive messages from Spirit before transmitting them, prompting some pedants to label their work as mediumistic rather than simply channeled information due to this very nuanced second delay between receiving and transmitting the information.

While many passages in my book are inspired by my guides, who assist me in keeping things moving smoothly and simply expressing these phenomena, I am also aware that, as a result of decades of work and study in this field, I occasionally share my own personal knowledge with them, and they simply inspire me in the most effective and correct manner.

They do direct my thoughts and words in this manner, but I get the clear sensation that, in some cases, I am serving as a conduit rather than a channel.

Again, we humans are continually seeking to categorize and construct absolutes around events that appear to contradict this method at times.

When we interact with guides, it is vital that they communicate with us in a creative, playful, and responsive manner, particularly in the early stages of our interactions. As your relationship matures and your mutual confidence grows, you may begin to accumulate items that you consider sophisticated.

To begin, we must establish that there is a distinct energy and awareness attempting to communicate with you, and we must then continue testing and experimenting with this consciousness until you are convinced that developing the communication channel is safe, useful, and beneficial to humanity.

The following meditation will take you on a journey to meet a guide or guardian angel, whichever you like. This guardian angel or guide interacts with you via a symbol and conveys an important message.

When you practice this meditation on a regular basis, preferably daily, you will build a personal symbolic language with your guide, allowing you to communicate with your guide as well as others.

If you wish to commit enough time to the long-term research and development of your gifts, I strongly suggest you keep a meditation journal. It might also be a blank-paged journal in which you scribble and record your experiences as you chat and interact with your mentors.

You can recognize big trends, continue to gather symbols that your guide can use to communicate with you and keep track of any noteworthy wins that strengthen your belief in the truth of your own experiences.

The crucial thing is that you properly test your strategy and enjoy the entire process. Make a conscious effort not to be unduly impatient for results but rather to appreciate that each blunder is a crucial step toward determining how well your abilities operate.

In addition to being a medium, angel intuitive, and channel, I am also a psychological development tutor. As a psychic development educator, I teach people how to develop their intuition and connect with their guides and angels, as well as how to enhance their psychological skills and feel inspired when working on creative projects.

While working as a psychological development educator and on my own personal growth journey, I've picked up a few tips for exploring and improving our ability to speak with our guides, teachers, and other creatures in the invisible worlds.

I hope you find them useful as you continue your studies and that you make a commitment to staying in touch with your guides so that they can always steer your work with their knowledge and love in the kindest and noblest way possible.

Request Connection Information

However, you'd be amazed how many people claim to want to work with their angels and guides but never seek assistance. It's almost as if these great, always-present teachers aren't listening to what they're saying. Our ever-patient teachers, on the other hand, are always present in the unseen realms, waiting for the signal that we choose to connect with them and always monitoring us, without judgment, as we navigate life.

Our angels and guides will never interfere with or undermine our free will, and they will always collaborate with us. Of course, they will continue to lead us unconsciously, but in ways that will help us improve our lives and prevent us from taking risks while also adhering to rigid norms that will allow us to live freely and put the lessons we have learned throughout our lives into practice.

If you actually want to build a conscious connection with your guides, allowing you to interact with them and receive their responses, as well as use their inspired counsel to help others, it may be good to ask them directly and purposefully what they are willing to do. This will help you to deliver a more powerful and unambiguous message that they will be able to respond to and act on. Make your inquiries as loud as possible to avoid confusion between your brief inquiries and your sincere desire to communicate outside the assumption field.

As a result, your angels and guides will be able to manifest much more forcefully in your life. Finally, when they believe you are absolutely prepared to receive their presence, they willfully and thoroughly reveal themselves.

It's wonderful that these connections may be sensed and comprehended. They improve people's lives simply by being present, and every interaction with one is a stimulating and satisfying experience in and of itself.

If you believe it will be beneficial, you may make your request through prayer. You can create a spiritual setting by settling into a comfortable position and lighting a white candle. Allow yourself to be guided into this sacred area by focusing on the highest vibrations of love and service to others. This is why the question is so crucial and answering it is one of the most crucial things we can do. In your diary, make a note that your guides will respond to any encounters you have during meditation or in your regular life in the days following your request for contact.

Meditation

If you only had one job, meditation would be the only way to communicate with your inner direction. Meditation is the most time-tested and traditional means of connecting with higher intelligence and nurturing and maintaining these relationships throughout time.

Our guides and angels communicate with us and with them on a daily basis. We are unaware of the vast majority of these meetings because our mentors and teachers are typically on distinct planes of reality. Despite the fact that these worlds exist only above the physical plane, they can only be visited via a doorway in the superconscious mind that is accessible via the conscious mind.

Many of us are entirely oblivious of this huge area of infinite possibilities, but our connection to it continuously showers us with flashes of insight and intuition. On occasion, they enter our consciousness through gaps and crevices. As ludicrous as that may appear, I'm sure we've all had the experience of reaching for the phone and then decided it wasn't a good idea at the time. Finally, we realized that if we had picked it up right away, we would have missed something else going on at the same time, which ended up saving the day in an unusual way.

Alternatively, we may be forced to take a left rather than a right, only to stumble into an old buddy we haven't seen in years.

When we meditate, we can access an infinite amount of unconscious information and begin to bring it into waking awareness. The barriers between dimensions begin to dissolve, and the better we are at shifting our energies from the third to the fourth dimension, where our angels, guides, and instructors reside, the faster this process will occur.

When we are fully awake and cognizant, we dedicate a significant percentage of our energy to controlling and learning from our physiological experiences. With its demands, distractions, and day-to-day practical problems, the world may appear to be all-consuming.

When we close our eyes, the brain creates alpha brain waves, allowing us to achieve a deep level of relaxation. In this approach, we can progressively become aware of a variety of parallel dimensions to the physical plane, and as a result, have access to communications and delicate interactions that occur frequently but are generally undetectable in such areas.

When we turn off the third dimension's noises and focus our attention within, giving ourselves the time and space to listen to what is happening, those other dimensions become more accessible, and our relationship with them develops deeper with each visit.

It takes time, effort, and consistent practice to build these connections, and meditation is the most basic and powerful method available. Doris Stokes is an established medium in her own right. Doris Stokes, one of my favorite mediums, used to meditate and communicate with her spiritual guidance on a daily basis.

As we practice meditation, our ability to calm our thoughts, activate our inner ears, and hear these other realities grow. With practice, our ability to listen grows, and the voices of our guides and teachers become stronger and clearer.

Disconnect Your Vibrations

What does it mean to say that we want to enhance our vibration, and why is this so critical? One reason for this is that when our vibration improves, we raise our frequency to that of love, which benefits both ourselves and the planet. It also improves the flow of our lives and all of our connections, and it motivates us to live from our hearts in beautiful and delightful ways, as well as to impact the vibrations of everyone in our immediate vicinity.

Chapter 25:
Psychic Empaths and Society

Favorites aren't psychic. It is not a privilege that just a few people enjoy. Psychological competency encompasses a wide variety of abilities. This could imply that you believe you can be summoned to read other people's emotions and thoughts. Furthermore, scientists have revealed that genes and childhood significantly impact whether or not a talent develops naturally.

Ancestry

The family history of a person is considered to play a big role in determining whether or not a child would be psychic. Furthermore, if shamans were used in the communities, the shaman's progeny should be prepared to take over after his father dies.

Shari Cohn began her research in Scotland by examining changes between residences in the highlands and the western islands. She discovered that many families appear to have the power of second vision, retrocognition (seeing into the past), and precognition in lonely areas where psychic ability is non-existent (seeing the future). Cohn examined 238 people and discovered that many of them possessed psychological aptitude. She also mentioned that women with twins or who are related to twins are more likely to be psychic and mentally intuitive.

Furthermore, Cohn's research found that families with psychic abilities and a belief in them benefited from a long line of psychics. Sylvia Wright also confirmed this connection. Children's psychic abilities are frequently suppressed in homes that do not believe in or cultivate them. Children who grow up in loving and supporting households, on the other hand, develop extraordinary psychic powers.

A psychic informed a sociologist about a time when she was a child and alerted her mother to the presence of a man in her room. "What is his name?" her mother said.

Another clairvoyant stated that her grandmother assisted her in improving her gaming skills by hiding a key in her house and instructing her to "be the key, then see where you are."

Stress and childhood trauma also have an impact on the development of psychic abilities. According to a researcher who spent years interviewing psychics and mediums, nearly every person examined had experienced some kind of personal catastrophe throughout their childhood. The University of Chicago discovered comparable outcomes in psychic interviews. Children who are exposed to family strife or have a troubled relationship with one of their parents (the father is more likely to develop psychic powers than the mother) develop psychic abilities, according to the study. Surprisingly, these participants were significantly happier with their current lives than the national average. The study revealed that psychic abilities were associated with rigorous education but had no effect on adult satisfaction.

It's scientifically known as "use it or lose it." Each of us is born with hundreds of thousands of brain cells. These cells will die as we age if they are not utilized. Everything you experience as a child before the age of ten has an impact on the type of brain cells that are preserved. Cell development determines how the brain organizes itself. If a child possesses psychic abilities, the brain is stimulated to utilize additional brain cells, allowing the child to grow. If the cells are not utilized, they will die.

Proteins are produced when genes, cells, and neurons are activated. When a child is encouraged and assisted in developing psychic abilities, and a penchant for the psychic, new pathways in the brain are formed that allow for development. A well-cared-for, intelligent child's brain will continue to develop until up to roughly 11 or 12 years old.

Psychologists have investigated the causes of trauma. When children are traumatized, their minds typically become disconnected from their surroundings. It will redirect the infant's attention away from conscious reality in order to protect him. Dissociating the brain allows it to adapt to different realities, potentially even distinct universes, places, and epochs. Several witnesses to traumatic events as youngsters have claimed sensations that occurred outside of their bodies. One of these psychics experienced physical attacks on a near-daily basis. Despite knowing and seeing what was going on, she stated that she would not hear or feel anything during the abuse. As a result, she would be forced to leave.

Another study looked at alcoholic or drug-addicted youngsters to investigate how early stress influenced their psychological abilities. The group frequently discusses their reactions to other people's beliefs, particularly those of their parents. According to one participant in a 1999 study, he frequently got home without knowing where his mother was. Despite the fact that he had never seen his mother before, he was aware of her current position as soon as he entered the house. He schooled himself to understand her feelings and moods so he would be able to recognize when she became illogical or unstable. Psychic empathy is the ability to experience and perceive another person's pain and emotions. Adolescents develop this as a self-protection tactic rather than disassociation.

Other psychiatric markers include whether a child was born to authoritarian, demanding, or abusive parents, such as loving parents who wanted perfect obedience. Other signs and symptoms include the loss of a mother for a small child, significant difficulties or malformations that necessitate recurrent fixes, and bipolar parents. A combination of stress and family history increases the possibility of psychic ability.

According to studies, psychic trends can occur in anyone, but they usually require a trigger, such as early trauma, a traumatic event, or family history. This should happen before the age of ten to thicken the frontal lobe and allow for the formation of synapses and neurons. The sole exception is if the child is exceptionally brilliant and has a high IQ;

in this case, the child must wait until the front lobe has gone through 12 modifications.

Consider your childhood. How did you spend your days? As a child, did you have to deal with a lot of stress? Did one of your parents die while you were a kid? Have you ever been in an extraordinary circumstance when you could tell something was going to happen or see things that others couldn't see? You're now looking for ways to improve your life and discover how to live more successfully using psychic abilities.

Chapter 26:
Psychic Empaths and Spiritual Awakening

The term "spiritual awakening" refers to a spiritual path of self-discovery and growth. Dreams, visions, spiritual experiences, and a range of physical events can all function as unconscious reawakening catalysts. The way an individual's feelings shift from person to person is determined by whether they have an open mind or a closed heart.

While there are numerous types of awakenings, each person's experience is unique based on their prior experiences and current circumstances. Here are some examples:

The Suffering Soul's Awakening

Soul awakening refers to the sensation of slipping away from the body after death and remaining connected to it for an extended amount of time or till death. It's also a time for spiritual rebirth. When a soul's physical body decays, it has the ability to evolve into a spiritual being. This change happens about a year after death.

The resurrection of the Spirit

A painful experience can cause a spiritual awakening, leading to a new understanding of one's life purpose or the path that one's soul is supposed to travel. Individuals who have had a spiritual awakening are more likely to want personal growth as a result of the experience. A person's spiritual awakening may spark a greater interest in spirituality and personal development, leading to the acquisition of books and attendance at classes on these subjects.

A spiritual awakening is a period of change or transition in one's life that occurs as a result of a substantial emotional struggle or catastrophe. Fear or guilt do not paralyze a person who accepts personal responsibility for their actions and the ability to decide the course of their life. Despite the fact that it may be intimidating to some, many people learn to utilize it in their personal and professional lives.

Excessive fury or grief may result in spiritual insight. When a person is overtaken by an overwhelming emotion, such as rage or grief, the mind usually acts as though it is going through the same thing. An overpowering emotional event, such as despair, fury, or a significant life event that precipitates a spiritual crisis, frequently causes a person to spiritually awaken. This can be a very difficult and stressful procedure for the individual, but it can also result in a whole new life experience they never believed imaginable.

Kundalini Re-Awakening

Kundalini awakening happens when a person feels powerful physical and spiritual sensations as a result of Kundalini's rising energy. It is supposed to occur more frequently when you are agitated, meditating, or engaging in other chakra-related activities.

Kundalini awakening is distinguished by a powerful sensation of warmth that begins near the base of the spine and gradually increases in intensity as it ascends the spine and throughout the body. People have said that they are experiencing a surge of energy throughout their bodies and that they need to exercise on occasion to relieve tension. Shaking, intense heat or cold, body vibrations or spasms, tiny ears, vision, and physiological experiences are among physical signs of Kundalini rising. This might be frightening for the individual experiencing it, and it is sometimes considered a medical emergency. The Kundalini awakening experience is intended to be pleasant; some people report feeling a strong sense of love and peace, while others report receiving a vision or message from a spirit or God; however, in approximately 10% of cases, the experience can lead to Kundalini Syndrome, a neurological condition. If Kundalini energy is not channeled, it can become neurotic, delusory, or even violent. If the crisis persists, the individual may require institutionalization and may turn suicidal.

Kundalini awakening is a yoga concept as well as a significant spiritual endeavor that requires the guidance of a competent instructor. Several accounts have surfaced throughout this time period of people being hurt or even murdered as Kundalini "attempts" to awaken spontaneously.

Most people think that Kundalini energy is dormant at birth and may be reawakened through meditation, yoga, and energy work. The majority of Kundalini awakening literature recommends proceeding slowly and gradually as your energy moves through the chakras, periodically monitoring your energy levels and adjusting your activities as appropriate. In this manner, you can ensure that your body can absorb the increased energy and prepare for the profound spiritual experiences that will accompany Kundalini awakening.

The awakening of one's third eye

Many individuals in the Western world are experiencing a period of consciousness regeneration, which is defined by the birth of fresh and innovative ideas, which typically materialize as societal revolution or spiritual enlightenment. We have experienced this occurrence from the Age of Enlightenment (early 18th century) to the Great French Revolution and even today's human awakening (21st century). In popular culture, this shift is referred to as "the waking of the third eye" or "the metamorphosis." The Third-Eye Awakening is a powerful and positive energy event that broadens collective consciousness and enables it to confront unresolved negative emotions and events. It also symbolizes the end of a cycle and the start of a new epoch, from which a new paradigm emerges. This can occur in individual lives as well as across entire countries, cultures, and civilizations.

In 1789, there was the French Revolution, followed by years of conflict and misery throughout the world. To paraphrase Don Quixote, we've seen people become more aware of their spirituality in recent years, such as the Sgt. Pepper's Lonely Hearts Club Band or the San Francisco Renaissance. In addition, a new generation of lightworkers and awakened folks is actively elevating Gaia and humanity, which is excellent. Because the vast majority of people are going on spiritual growth journeys, the "Shift" is at an all-time high right now. It all begins with a growing interest in spirituality and self-discovery, as well as a belief in a greater power at work in their lives. The fact that many individuals are embracing religion, which was previously absent from their lives, is significant evidence of this shift.

Spiritual factors that promote enlightenment

Discovering one's spiritual nature can be a challenging and complicated journey. However, returning to the underlying notion of spiritual enlightenment. Spiritual awakening is not a common occurrence, despite the fact that it has occurred to many people throughout history. It still happens, albeit less frequently. As a result, what causes spiritual ascension? Is it feasible to discover certain variables that contribute to a person's spiritual awakening and assist them in recognizing their inherent spirit? Continue reading for more information!

The majority of people do not experience any spiritual awakening in their lifetimes. According to some assessments, many people today appear to have lost contact with their spiritual selves or even the realization that they have one.

Those who have experienced spiritual awakening, on the other hand, have discovered that they have a soul and have learned to cherish the significance of this in their lives. Their minds are expanded, and many of them begin to seek greater importance in their lives than they previously did. Spiritual awakening is defined as the soul's eyes opening – or, at the very least, the soul being recognized after a long time of denial – and is often accompanied by a sense of enlightenment or nirvana. Furthermore, many awakened people realize that their physical body is not the only thing in their existence and how everything, both physically and spiritually, fits together. Spiritual awakening is a wonderful thing that can occur in a variety of ways. The majority of individuals struggle to accept that they are spiritually enlightened and that their lives transcend beyond their physical bodies. Individuals who have this experience, on the other hand, usually find that they begin to perceive the world in a whole new light, and as a result, they obtain a new understanding of reality.

The waking process is fascinating, and it frequently results in dramatic changes in a person's daily routine. A change in your pay – which is usually the outcome of your company's overall performance – and a difference in your attitude toward your employment are two examples. To name a few features, a spiritual awakening sometimes involves much more than simply viewing oneself as spiritually awakened; it also necessitates some knowledge of one's position in the greater cosmos, as well as the belief that the universe has an interior soul. Many people are taken aback by spiritual awakening since it is frequently difficult to understand at first. This is a once-in-a-lifetime chance that the vast majority of people will never have. Those who are aware of it rarely behave in ways that suggest they have attained spiritual enlightenment. As a result, the vast majority of people are completely oblivious of the process, which they only discover after a significant period of time has elapsed.

This is because awakened people frequently reflect on their lives, perplexed by what has transpired and why they have done what they have done. Prior to awakening, their lives appeared to be a dream, and when they awoke, they realized there was more going on – that divine energy was present in their lives – that they were awake. As a result, awakening can be challenging at first, but the work is well worth it.

The Spiritual Enlightenment Trigger

This is a relatively new area of spirituality and awakening research and literature that has evolved in the last few years. It is yet unknown who these triggers are and what they do. Some believe they are the source of spiritual enlightenment, while others believe they should be avoided. The concept of "spiritual triggers" is novel and difficult to grasp. Any external encounter that shatters a person's vision of reality, rendering their current belief system ineffective in dealing with the issue, is referred to as a spiritual trigger.

People who are resistive to spiritual influences are also resistant to spiritual enlightenment. They consider their own and others' opposition as proof that the rest of the world is incapable of obtaining enlightenment. On a more fundamental level, this results in a dreadful sense of immobility. This notion is exemplified by Michael Murphy's Ph.D. research into the composition of spiritual awakenings. He discovered that approximately half of the pupils had experienced significant religious decline or deterioration throughout their lives. Those who do not deteriorate, he claims, are either born resistant to change or have formed beliefs that change is not necessary for survival. The two lines of inquiry, spiritual awakening and spiritual awakening-related decline, do not have mutually exclusive findings.

Many people feel that well-known and, in some cases, inevitable spiritual triggers characterize the spiritual awakening process. This position is supported by the premise that the concept of reality is simply too rigid to change in the absence of an intervening event in one's life. People who are affected by this emotion are more likely to avoid the things that trigger their feelings. As a result, it may resolve to remain in its current religious and spiritual community as long as possible until a triggering event occurs. This is analogous to the notion of Buddhism's diminishing capacity to acquire new information, as evidenced by its refusal to do so.

Spiritual awakening, according to those who believe in its importance, is unavoidable. This is because there are no exceptions to what causes something to happen, such as how many times a person has been exposed before it occurs. This belief is supported by the lack of evidence indicating the existence of such an exception.

It is vital to remember that spiritual awakening is a novel concept that can be difficult to grasp at first. People who have undergone a spiritual awakening typically have a better grasp of themselves than they had previously. It is possible for people to change their behavior by perceiving their lives as if they were unfolding in front of their eyes rather than in the future. As a result, spiritual awakening and insights may have an impact on one's daily life.

Spiritual awakening is undoubtedly a wonderful thing, but it may also be extremely difficult to live with. Most people are unaware of this process throughout their lives, and they frequently discover that they have been spiritually awakened as a result of a life-changing incident. Their perspective on life shifts and spiritual awakenings frequently provide a lot of fresh information and understanding.

After all, because spiritual awakening is difficult to acclimate to, many people dismiss it as a myth or a fairy tale. Individuals who are experiencing it, on the other hand, are intensely aware that something out of the ordinary is happening. When you open your soul, you not only learn but also realize how much more important life may be.

You must decide what spiritual awakening means in your life and how to proceed. After all, awakening frequently demonstrates that there is more to life than meets the eye or that everything happens for a reason.

Chapter 27:
Things that Will Stop you From Enlightenment

A variety of things could prevent you from becoming spiritually enlightened. There are numerous methods for gaining anything by chance, ranging from mental to physical, or from moving too quickly to moving too slowly.

Overcoming Physical Difficulties

Our bodies are not always prepared for spiritual awakening, which is an unfortunate reality. In some cases, this has been connected to an autoimmune condition, but not in all. Meditation, however, may not always be possible due to a high level of daily anxiety. You will reach a point in your healing when you can accept spiritual awakening above all else, but that moment may not be right for you right now, which is just great. A rapid waking can be dangerous in some situations, so always go at a pace that appears natural and stress-free based on your experience and needs.

Things are experienced in a too intense or quick fashion.

Chakras naturally clog over time and can be easily opened, cleaned, and realigned. Those who have had a Kundalini awakening experience can awaken considerably faster than those who have not or are severely hampered. If you do, you will almost surely have a powerful experience right away, which may be too intense due to the quickness with which the transition occurs. If you don't rush things and continue to create more intense and rapid development than predicted, you should at the very least try to meditate every other day. Working with a mentor or guru also provides a lot of advantages. Despite widespread skepticism regarding these types of healing and awakening connections, your sensitivity qualifies you as an excellent teacher, mentor, or simply a sympathetic listener.

Some foods don't aid in awakening

Even though it appears to some to be excessive, your diet may occasionally hinder you from waking up (and I'd like to imagine that this "some" group is largely meat-eaters). By making a few modest tweaks, you may be able to speed up the waking process. Begin by eating fewer processed meals and more veggies and fruits. If you're having problems getting started, try reducing your weekly meal intake by one or two meals. Begin cautiously and pay attention to your feelings and physical reactions to the activity. If you get a positive response, keep tweaking your method.

You're focusing your attention on the wrong part of your body.

In other circumstances, spiritual awakening difficulties are caused by an inability to concentrate, which can be readily solved by shifting one's meditation focus. If you meditate by closing your eyes and focusing your attention on your head (or third eye), you've found the cause of the problem (as most people do). To begin spiritual awakening, you must first focus on your heart, stomach, and intestines. Kundalini thrives in a healthy environment, and focusing all of your healthy attention on your third eye will take you far beyond the intestine, where spirituals first meet, to a far higher level. Consider how the spirit will pass through you and how you will prepare your body. For the most part, take deep abdominal breaths and pay attention to how your state of mind changes throughout your meditations.

Your body knows your brain, but not vice versa.

This goal is attainable, but it will necessitate some physical work on your part. The link to yoga is important in this scenario since it can help you ignite your kundalini. Through movement and attention to the body, Kundalini yoga, in particular, aids in the removal of obstacles from the chakras. Throughout your journey, you must maintain a strong balance of mind-body talents. Otherwise, you'll be in a state of internal struggle for the foreseeable future.

Having a gloomy or disagreeable temperament

To some extent, awakening Kundalini can help with mood and emotional disorders, but you must first get there. Your elevated mood and emotional imbalances are most likely impeding your ability to perceive a clear path forward in your awakening journey. Check your assumptions! Take note of how you're feeling! Consider how you normally feel! If you can shift these ideas and moods in any manner, you will see a huge boost in your kundalini practice in a short amount of time. While it may appear difficult, demanding, or perplexing at this time, if you can rise above exhausting thoughts and feelings, you will find your kundalini rising in response.

Past trauma, often known as post-traumatic stress disorder (PTSD), is simply too powerful to avoid.

When we see (or are currently experiencing) traumas, we frequently form blocks in our chakras that grow so strong and pervasive that we are unable to guide ourselves through our own awakenings. That is simply a fact of life with no positive or negative consequences. If you are experiencing this sensation, please contact us right away since great and life-changing hope is accessible to you. It simply implies that your previous experiences have given you the ability to act on your own. Depending on your circumstances, it may be good to discuss your experiences with a friend, a lover, a guard (on this or another plane), or a therapist. If you are unable to speak with others, are hesitant to share your grief with others, or believe you have no one else with whom to share your experience, you should get treatment. Remove it from your system! Get this disgusting beast out of here! If you create anything or have a conversation about something, your Kundalini will rise swiftly.

Positive signs, amazing experiences, and delight are not always there. Change them, or you will lose your ability to endure more Kundalini action. This is an awful situation, but it almost certainly means that some people will continue to sleep as a result of their own reality tests.

Furthermore, as the kundalini travels through the neck, third eye, and head chakras, a person becomes more aware of their divinity (prior to the open chakras flowing freely). For some, this level of awareness may be terrifying or unsettling. Some people are simply unwilling to seize this opportunity. To overcome feelings of rejection, build an unusual level of openness and acceptance toward yourself, the divine, and others if you find yourself in a similar scenario.

You've almost certainly interacted with someone who attempted to convey their awakening to those closest to them but was unable or unable to accept community assistance. You may have heard that if your Kundalini awakens, you will lose control over your friends and family. It doesn't happen very often, but if it does, don't be quick to spread the news just yet, especially if you're with close friends or family.

Allow the Kundalini to ascend in the vicinity of these people.

1. As you advance along your waking journey, you will see a rise in your attractiveness. It goes without saying that if you keep the proper balance of hope and concentration, you will quickly attract the right kind of assistance.

3. The next time, you can repeat the process with friends and family, but this time employing a range of tactics.

4. You could even do away with the idea of a support group entirely and instead develop your own information community. There are numerous applications available for download that can assist you in improving your awakening by delivering useful thoughts and direction, and for some people, this information switch is sufficient to compensate for those in your surrounding environment.

You don't have access to a professor or a Guide to assist you.

While some people may be able to navigate their awakenings effectively on their own, others may benefit enormously from the instruction and support of a teacher or, at the absolute least, a mentor. If you're feeling lost and in need of guidance, my first suggestion is to find a kundalini yoga institution. See what comes up when you speak with a teacher at the school. If you want to meet in person, seek kundalini chat groups online or inquire about meditation instructors at your local metaphysical store. Never fight on your own. Allow Kundalini to direct your trust in order to attract those who can assist you in growing.

Unfavorable environments for recovery

If you desire to awaken, some settings, whether in your home, job, natural environment, or elsewhere, will prevent you from doing so. Someone will say something dumb every now and again that will lead you to lose your train of thought. You may also be exposed to chemicals that cause your pineal gland to calcify without your knowledge, such as when working in a dangerous environment. You should trust your intuition in this scenario. If you're not comfortable where you're meditating or performing yoga, try relocating. If you're terrified of who you are or what you want to accomplish, go somewhere safe to hide until you're ready to face the world. Seek treatment if you feel threatened by who you are and what you want to do. You are not required to do this process under duress, and you are certainly not required to do so in a hazardous setting.

Chapter 28:
The Effect of Awakening

We become more aware of our own feelings as a result of our spiritual awakening. That is the beginning of everything. We are now in a position to evaluate our own actions. It usually occurs in the following sequence:

Feelings of unhappiness and emptiness.

This could be the result of a traumatic occurrence in your life. The reason for your sadness or uneasiness is frequently hidden from you. Divorce, a traumatic event, death, cancer, or other life-changing events are common triggers. Whatever occurs, you may get isolated from the rest of the world, which will be harmful to your health.

The surrounding environment has shifted.

As a result of this awakening, you may be able to see through the lies used against you. You're currently dissatisfied and irritated with your surroundings. You may be angry and sad at the same time, creating the impression that you are on an emotional roller coaster. That is how your mind works. The spiritual enlightenment of a person is preceded by a series of events known as phases. When this occurs, some people are aware, while others are not. The following are symptoms that you are on the verge of spiritual awakening:

You avoid folks who are negative.

If you find yourself giggling, passing judgment, or engaging in other exaggerated behavior, avoid these folks. After a certain point, you'll realize that it's no longer quite as large.

Developing a near-perfect intuition.

When it comes to other people, you'd rather focus on their deeds than their words. Simply make sure you're paying attention and don't tell anyone what you've seen. People with manipulative tendencies will strive to modify the situation.

Validation isn't necessary. You desire more alone and introspective time. As a result, social media will gradually fade from your life. You'll notice that you're no longer relying on social media to gauge your popularity; instead, you'll feel comfortable in your own skin. If you are fortunate enough to experience spiritual awakening, it can be a great experience. A spiritual awakening can dramatically enhance someone's life, happiness, health, and prosperity in a short amount of time. This type of situation is not always simple to deal with, but if you have a spiritual awakening, the positive impacts on your life will last a lifetime. As you ascend and descend the stairs, you will understand how wonderful the experience may be, and you will not want to miss it. Many individuals find spiritual awakening to be a tough and complicated process to grasp. As a result, people may struggle to understand what this phenomenon means to them. Spiritual awakening is a unique journey that varies from individual to person. It could be as simple as shedding a few tears while watching a movie or as sophisticated as observing nature and regaining strength. Awakenings of various kinds can endure for days, weeks, or even decades. Others may struggle to understand spiritual awakening since it looks to them to be a one-time, transient experience.

Increased chakra activity is the most common type of spiritual awakening. It's likely that you'll feel like you're flying. As a result of their experience, some people refer to this as "coming to life" or "experiencing life for the first time." This type of awakening lasts only a few minutes, and most people are immediately aware of it. It's a sign that you're reconnecting with your actual self and accepting your own identity. When people develop a greater understanding of the spiritual realm and how it operates, they experience a different form of awakening than they expected. People may be enthralled rather than delighted by this new revelation, especially if it relates to their own psychic powers. You may be ecstatic to be a part of a spiritual community and feel inspired to continue on your spiritual path. There's a good possibility you believe you have a goal to accomplish and that you're looking forward to enjoying the scenery along the way. You may get the impression that you have been awakened to a magnificent truth that will offer you endless joy. When you first discover or develop your psychic skills, you go through a spiritual awakening. This normally happens later in life, after a person has had the opportunity to get familiar with the spiritual realm and fulfill their full potential. Individuals frequently develop abilities that they previously lacked during this phase of waking, such as the ability to predict the future or read the emotions of those around them. It is also possible to hear or see unauthentic things. When they find their potential to seek out energy bigger than themselves, they may get bewildered and begin to doubt their abilities.

Spiritual awakenings are more prevalent among those who meditate or study spirituality. This is the most prevalent sort of awakening since it is initiated by people who desire to connect with their spirituality. Your psychic abilities can be both perplexing and entertaining. While your visions or dreams may overwhelm you, you can also consider them as an opportunity to enhance your spiritual understanding of the circumstance. Individuals who practice meditation and spirituality, on the other hand, may experience the inverse effect. They are generally calm and quiet for the first few days or weeks but gradually become restless or uncomfortable. People believe their lives are meaningful or significant at this time, but the emotion fades rapidly, and the event no longer feels spiritual. Some people claim to have had extremely beneficial experiences as a result of their spiritual awakening. It's likely that the prospect of making a life-changing discovery will pique your attention. They may have a strong sense of purpose in life and are steadfast in their determination to overcome hurdles. Instead of increasing your self-awareness, you may become more confused and insecure.

Many individuals believe that experiencing a spiritual awakening at a certain age will change their lives forever. Children may struggle to understand the significance of their experience as a result of this energy fluctuation. If you've experienced spiritual awakening, you'll realize that the energy around you is radically different from the energy you've been exposed to your entire life. It's possible that you're feeling the entirety of your being for the first time. You can also be aware that you are on a journey and that there are several things that need to be completed.

Others, on the other hand, may have to wait years, if not decades, before seeing any benefits. Some may assume that this experience is over and that it no longer exists in reality. Others, on the other hand, see this as the start of something far larger. A multitude of variables influence your spiritual enlightenment. There's no doubting that your previous and life experiences have an impact on this process. Many people begin meditating or practicing spirituality when they feel confined or unhappy in their lives. They usually start with yoga or meditation practices and quickly understand their connection to both personal and universal energy. Prolonged meditation and skill development help you obtain a better understanding of yourself and the spiritual world. These individuals may be drawn to spiritual teachings or lectures that explain how the spiritual realm operates in the present. Maybe you want a more intense spiritual experience to better understand the connections between the physical and spiritual realms. They can, however, be turned around. As your confidence in meditation or spirituality grows, you may realize that you require greater stability and meaning in your life. They can now focus their efforts on a single life objective, such as obtaining work, marrying, or starting a family. This will have an effect on the procedure depending on the type of spiritual awakening experiences you've had.

Pros

As a result, many people are skeptical about the benefits of spiritual awakening since they are unaware of what they would get as a result. However, knowing that this form of spiritual awakening benefits all parts of one's life is reassuring. It enables you to develop a deeper understanding of yourself and the impact of your actions on people around you. Furthermore, many individuals believe it is long-term helpful to one's physical health. The following are only a handful of the benefits of spiritual awakening.

You will have a greater understanding of yourself.

When you have a spiritual awakening, you begin to see that your previous expectations may not always mirror reality or even the source of your happiness. After experiencing spiritual awakening, you will learn that your potential is far more than you realize and that you have far more capacity than you realize.

As a result, your confidence will grow.

Self-doubt can prevent us from attaining our goals in a variety of aspects of our lives, but when we believe in ourselves, we are unstoppable. Self-assured people are more inclined to feel good about themselves and do what they desire.

You'll realize you have a bigger role to play in everything.

We all enter and depart this planet on our own, but a significant portion of life can only be lived as part of a family, community, or other groups in between. If you experience a spiritual awakening, you will learn that your actions have far more implications than you realize and that you must consider how your actions may affect others before acting.

It will make your life more enjoyable.

Although the world is a fantastic playground, we may easily lose sight of it as we grow engaged in each tiny drama. A spiritual awakening, on the other hand, may offer you a new and deeper appreciation for how lovely the world is and how fortunate you are to live in it. This newly discovered appreciation will make you feel more grateful for the time you have left on this earth.

It will greatly simplify your life.

We all face obstacles at some point in our life, and when we don't know how to handle them, it's natural to become frustrated with our situations. Those who have experienced a spiritual awakening, on the other hand, learn that facing problems can actually make you wiser and isn't as frightening as you might think. When you comprehend this, your fear will dissipate, and you will be less likely to perish in perilous situations.

It increases your capacity to empathize.

In addition to your admiration for the planet, you will develop a greater sense of compassion for the people around you, as well as a better knowledge of how their actions influence you and others. This knowledge can help you acquire more patience and understanding, which will make life easier for others around you.

This increases your motivation to take action.

In a world where people frequently fail to see the value of the things they are passionate about, it may be difficult to find meaning in all you do. If you've had a spiritual awakening, you'll see that love, like everything else, has intrinsic value and must be exchanged on occasion. That's when you begin to notice the things that actually make you happy.

It can help you preserve your health during difficult circumstances.

While it may be difficult to remain cool in stressful situations, spiritual awakenings can help us put our own thoughts into context. They may offer us a sense of tranquility and tranquility, allowing us to maintain constant contact with the rest of the group.

Because the world is filled with people who are hurting and feeling alone, it is critical that you reach out to others while you are going through a difficult time. However, as your spiritual awareness grows, you will recognize that the people in your life are part of a larger family, which will increase their value in your eyes.

When we are down and out, our faith may be put to the test as our lives get increasingly difficult, and we wonder why we were dealt such a bad hand. If, on the other hand, you have a spiritual awakening, you may find that your faith is strengthened as you realize that everything is part of God's plan and that everything has an answer.

It could help you keep a healthy lifestyle.

When people are unhappy with their life or are worried and anxious about themselves or others, they often turn to food for solace. If, on the other hand, you have a spiritual awakening, you will realize that your source of happiness is within you and that there is no reason to deny yourself these feelings by relying on food to get through life.

It's easy to lose sight of life's magnificent gift when we're anxious and wish things were different. After experiencing a spiritual awakening, you will understand that you have had one of the most magnificent experiences possible and that your life is full of wonder and potential.

Cons

Spiritual awakening is a life-changing experience that can be abrupt and disastrous in certain cases, but it can also be gradual and include direct contact with the Divine. It varies from religious conversion or being "born again" in that it is unrelated to a person's religious views. Consider the disadvantages of having a fully awakened state of consciousness:

You may feel bad about what you've done to help your spiritual development.

For example, someone may cause himself pain by opening up to another person and recognizing their own higher purpose. After acquiring enlightenment, a person is relieved of guilt for having experienced that dreadful emotion because he has already turned into a better person. Their craving for guilt has outpaced their understanding of their previous transgressions, and they have become ignorant to them. While this may appear to be liberating at first, the individual may come to realize that guilt was the instrument he used to learn and experience who he is and what his higher purpose is if he lacks it.

Knowing what others have been through but not knowing who they are is disappointing.

When a person is dissatisfied, they seek something more significant to fill the emptiness, which can result in the creation of legends and myths to fill the void, or it can lure them like a moth to a light bulb.

As a result, the individual loses all ties to their former self.

As a result of this, he develops an unhealthy connection to himself and considers living in a monastery and leading a spiritual lifestyle. This may have a particularly severe influence on persons who were once religious but are no longer clear about what religion is. Even while you're awake, achieving a balance between your prior and current states might be difficult.

Essentially, the concept of their majesty and brilliance has captured their attention.

This could result in an obsession that lasts as long as the experience does. This is a type of OCD that has the ability to cause more issues in a person's life than it solves. When a person is reawakened, they should not simply sit back and bask in the glory of their accomplishment. You must completely comprehend the significance of this experience in order to progress independently on your higher path.

The individual may believe that they are in a superior position.

This is a rather common occurrence as a result of awakening, not only because of the urge for self-validation but also because anyone who has had such a strong experience is naturally drawn to share it with others, even if they are not interested in hearing about it.

The individual feels ecstatic at the thought of being revived and believes they have attained "superhuman" status.

Individuals assume they have attained a higher level of realization than others, despite the fact that there is no such state of realization in reality. The ego can take over and convince a person that they are superior to others in a variety of ways. This is a fabricated sense of superiority in one's own talents rather than a genuine epiphany.

The individual has developed an obsessive fixation with the event in question.

They are unable to break free because they do not understand what it means to be spiritually awakened and how much effort it takes to maintain their new perspective on themselves. When someone strives to maintain this new consciousness and recognizes that others are not in the same condition as them, they become more demanding, critical, and negative than before.

The individual may become unduly dedicated to their higher purpose or enlightenment, isolating themselves from family and friends.

This has a lot of promise. If you devote your entire life to your greater purpose, you will believe that it is the only thing that matters and that everything else is a hindrance to achieving it. Because your waking experience left you feeling disconnected from others, a void in your life is likely to form, leading to loneliness.

Chapter 29:
Facets of Awakening

Seekers become aware of this aspect gradually or abruptly and observe its impact on their beliefs and perceptions of the environment in which they find themselves. Emotional or mental conceptions will no longer surprise or fool the searcher when his mental model collapses and is replaced by consciousness.

Our basic self-perception is inextricably tied to physical experiences and emotional responses. When we are upset, we express our feelings by saying "I" am angry. We identify with someone else's feelings when we feel sad for them. When you become conscious of your emotions, you stop defining yourself by them. You understand that emotions are essentially brain products with no long-term consequence or ability to influence a person's thinking or conduct.

When one awakens to the side of the mind, the distinction between thinking and consciousness becomes clear. At this point, the seeker is no longer deceived by the brain's output and recognizes that his ideas and sensations are distinct from his consciousness. Two examples are the seeker's ability to detect feelings and emotions mentally after thoroughly awakening without becoming entangled in them and the seeker's ability to monitor thoughts and emotions throughout one's life cycle without allowing them to cloud judgment.

The seeker is also conscious of his or her own ego and the part it plays in the human psyche at this time. It's also worth noting that most seekers will not fully comprehend the breadth and reach of their egos until that part of themselves is fully awakened.

When most people become aware of their own beliefs, they experience a dramatic transformation. This is not to say that the awakened individual is devoid of all emotions and sensations. It still elicits emotions such as rage, anger, envy, greed, lust, and guilt, among others, but instead of influencing a person's judgment, it is up to the individual to determine how much, if any, of his or her thoughts and emotions should have an impact.

All emotions become crucial instruments for the fully awakened individual, helping them to become conscious of unresolved wounds or traumas or to return to old conditioning.

The Various Facets of Oneself

Aspects of the searchers' ego gradually or suddenly become awake, and they develop a holistic awareness of their ego, which Buddhism identified and vanquished thousands of years ago. Science continues to lag behind the rest of the world in the modern era.

By perceiving one's own past and letting go of all attachments, the seeker can untangle their thinking and consciousness. As a result, the awakened individual no longer suffers in its entirety. This is because the awakened individual achieves a state of consciousness in which everything, including the current moment, is unreservedly welcomed without preference for one instant over another.

The newly awakened individual is capable of accepting complete responsibility for their entire existence and everything that transpires within it. They no longer hold individuals accountable for their earlier sadness because they understand that grief is the result of the ego. The awakened person no longer attempts to impose his or her beliefs on others, understanding that we are all making the best judgments we can at the time and that we are all responsible for our own learning and internal growth.

After integrating this new knowledge into daily life, the seeker typically loses all consciousness of his or her physical body (emotional, physical, and thought). They gain confidence and develop a strong and lasting feeling of self-worth. Your need for traditional kinds of connection has shifted, and you are no longer concerned with conforming or being "normal." You have the right to be yourself without requesting permission or consent from others, and you may do so even without their awareness.

The personality of the awakened seeker may endure subtle changes that are visible to people in his near surroundings. One prevalent misunderstanding in this area is that an awakened person's personality changes as a result of their waking or illumination; however, this is not the case here. Except for any character or personality traits that were unhealthy or did not help him along the journey to spiritual illumination in the previous stage, a fully awakened person will retain his or her former personality.

"Normal" society has vanished as a result of the need to fit in, the inherent habit of being politically correct or being subordinated to "normal" society. Rather than acting on ego, the seeker considers what is best for them and everyone else involved in any given situation. The seeker's search for happiness comes to an end on a regular basis because she realizes that nothing else can satisfy her.

The Spiritual Energy Face is a portrait of a person who possesses spiritual energy.

At its most fundamental, spiritual energy is universal energy that goes through and into the human body via a multitude of paths. When one recognizes the reality of spiritual energy, also known as Qi (chi), prana (prana), and chakras, physiological, mental, and spiritual shifts occur (or kundalini energy). Tai Chi, yoga, meditation, and tantra are some of the ancient techniques that can aid in the awakening of this energy, which, like any other awakening, can occur gradually or suddenly.

The Public Persona of Universal Consciousness

A global consciousness emanates from the wellspring of all things. This source is referred to by some as cosmic comprehension, while others refer to it as God, Allah, or the Great Spirit. It is impossible to be divorced from Universal Consciousness because human consciousness is derived from it, even if people only become fully conscious of it when they are fully conscious. Despite the fact that it resides outside of time and space, universal awareness can be found throughout the cosmos or all of space and time. It's best described as an unidentified intellect that underpins and directs the evolution of the physical universe as we know it.

As the human mind awakens to global knowledge, whether spontaneously or due to a massive internal explosion, it extends to cover the entire globe and even the stars. As a result of their efforts, a seeker may gain new insight into the essence of reality, as well as an infusion of love or knowledge. As a result of his or her awakening to another aspect, the seeker's conceptions of duality, such as good and evil, disintegrate completely, and he or she realizes that everything, including themselves, trees and rocks, planets and galaxies, and individual light particles and moments in time, is made up of pure love.

Aspirants who have fully awakened to this side of themselves know that their lives have no value or purpose. The seeker's passion for life, for everyone and everything in it springs from the depths of their hearts and reconnecting with everyone and everything offers them immense joy.

If they haven't already, a seeker will have entirely abandoned all fear of death at this point, and their sole attention will be on living in the present moment. When the physical body is seen as a way of conserving human knowledge, the dread of bodily loss becomes a constant cause of stress. Because the seeker recognizes that time and space are fundamentally human concepts, he or she identifies them as intellectual processes that assist people in analyzing change and their current circumstances.

The seeker finally realizes how everything in the cosmos is interconnected, how everything from trees to rocks to the human body is formed of the same substance, and how everything originates from the same place.

"Believing what you see," as the proverb goes, is one of those lines that serve to highlight what is perhaps the most significant fact that individuals have misunderstood at some point: that our environment is exactly what our eyes detect.

However, this is not the case. That is just untrue. This is completely false. According to science, the human eye can detect only 0.005% of all accessible wavelengths of energy, referred to as "visible light." According to astronomers and astrophysicists, just 4% of the universe is visible to the naked eye or any other contemporary technology, with the other 96 percent referred to as "dark matter."

Consider the atom, which is the fundamental unit of our universe. While it is largely assumed that our universe is 14 billion years old, some theories place the age much further back. Our bodies are entirely composed of carbon, nitrogen, and oxygen atoms that originated in stars older than our sun, in our galaxy, solar system, planet, and in the bodies of our ancestors and mothers.

Awakening's components can be assembled in any order, at any pace, and at any level relative to one another. Certain parts of awakening on one side can assist the seeker in awakening on the other, while others have no connection to each other.

Chapter 30:
Kickstart Your Psychic Journey

Meditation with a guide can assist you in developing psychic abilities.

Psychic meditation is similar to traditional meditation in that no special powers are required. It's a fantastic technique to connect with one's inner self while disconnecting from the outside world and honing one's talents. The distinction between regular and psychic meditation is that regular meditation seeks to produce a tranquil, stress-free mind, whereas psychic meditation seeks to cultivate psychic contact with the cosmos. Your intention, on the other hand, is to use psychic meditation to hone your intuitive senses and psychic skills.

We were all born with psychological qualities that we may all improve on a daily basis by meditating on a regular basis. You can either practice psychic meditation or develop mental powers as a psychic medium. Incorporating crystal stones, such as quartz, into our lives yields the finest outcomes since they have the power to heal our bodies while simultaneously increasing our spiritual energies. While holding the crystals in your hands or palms, you can meditate with an open mind and patience.

A Step-by-Step Guide to Psychic Meditation

1. <u>Make arrangements to be alone at a specified time and place.</u>
Before you begin, find a peaceful place where no one can annoy you and switch off all electrical equipment, including your phone. Make sure there are no children in the neighborhood so that your meditation can continue uninterrupted. You can delve deeper into your inner senses in a peaceful setting and have an absolutely great psychic contact.

Bring a pen and a notebook to your meditation session to keep track of your ideas and feelings. Although most people who meditate do so lying down, psychic meditation gurus encourage sitting in your favorite chair. Your palms resting on your chin represent your readiness to receive spiritual instruction.

2. Take note of your breathing rhythm.

You may focus only on your breathing when you close your eyes. This aids in slowing the frequency of brain waves, which is required to develop psychic skills. Inhale deeply via your nose and hold for three seconds, noticing how your hands expand on the inside of your tummy. Although it may appear difficult at first, remember that practice makes perfect. However, remember that you should never force yourself to do something you don't want to do.

Exhale three times through the lips and hold the air for three seconds. Check to see if all of the air you've inhaled has been completely discharged from your stomach. After a few minutes of using this breathing technique, you can slow down your breathing rate to achieve a calmer breathing pattern.

3. To protect yourself, define and explain your aim.

Before beginning a meditation session, you should have specific goals in mind. For defense against low-vibrational energy, contact your spirit guardians. This stage is critical because it helps you to work from a place of love, develops your psychic talents, and aids in the development of your psychic medium.

4. Be receptive to new knowledge.

You're now ready to hear information from your guide's spirits because you've raised your vibrations. Allow for the incorporation of imaginative and novel ideas into your thinking by keeping an open mind free of preconceived preconceptions. Begin by imagining everything that can lead to a possible opportunity. This signals to others that you are now receptive to new information. To name a few things, a light had been turned on, a book had been read, a flower had bloomed, and a door had been opened. These visuals will assist you in widening your awareness to spiritual understanding. Once you have these psychic powers, you should use them with caution and wisdom.

5. <u>Describe in detail your impressions.</u>

Visual images, physical sensations like pressure or pins and needles, emotional responses like sadness or happiness, and a few words or names with a strong sense of recognition may all arise in your mind's eye. Whatever comes to mind should be scribbled down.

6. <u>Never forget.</u>

Psychic meditation is employed because people's perceptions differ. No matter how terrifying the experience is, you should not be afraid. Furthermore, avoid forming visual predictions and instead let the images speak for themselves. If you're still perplexed, you can seek clarification from your mentors. With practice and time, this strategy gets simpler and faster, allowing you to adjust in and out quickly and without spending too much energy. As a result, you must be patient and persistent, as impatience may inhibit your psychic powers.

7. <u>How to End a Meditation Session Properly</u>

You were effective in incorporating new thoughts or information from your spirit guides into your consciousness. The final step is to double-check that you have finished your meditation. This is a vital stage that should not be missed; otherwise, you may have energy all day!

This can be accomplished by collecting information in the opposite direction from how you normally gather it. For example, if you have a candle in your mind, you can switch it off to see it go out. If you've seen the beginning of a book, you can estimate how it will end. Then, thank your spirit guides for their help and ask them to keep you safe from any negative energy.

After meditation, you should ground yourself to restore energy balance and eliminate any dazzling sensations that may have happened. Daily psychic meditation practice can help you improve and make your spiritual direction job easier and more fun.

Practices that will aid in the strengthening of your psychological link

Even if some people are born with mental abilities, everyone can learn new skills as an adult, so anybody can employ mental abilities. To increase our psychic skills, we simply need to learn how to connect with our intuition and bring it to life. These are just a few ideas on how to deepen your psychic connection.

1. Meditation methods

Meditation is a great method to unwind while simultaneously sharpening your focus and attention. It alleviates pain, decreases stress, and encourages relaxation and mental clarity. It is recommended that you meditate for 10-15 minutes each day to boost your body's vibration, which is vital for mental ability growth.

Meditation allows you to unwind and boost your energy vibration, which helps you develop your intuitive abilities and talents. As your tranquility and clarity rise, so will your ability to recognize the needs of those around you and learn more about yourself. Daily meditation can also help you develop a relationship with your spirit guides, who can help you gain psychological strength.

The greatest results are obtained by integrating crystal stones of your choice. Allow yourself to fully relax and interact with your soul by directing your attention above the level of your eyes. This can aid in the development and strengthening of psychic talents such as intuition, clairvoyance, and clairaudience.

2. Have confidence in yourself

Your level of self-assurance determines the development of psychic powers. The inner critic stifles the development of psychic powers. Never give up hope; only believe in yourself and your capacity to do your tasks on time and with as little effort as possible. Look for inspiration wherever you go, and learn about psychic development. You can even learn from and emulate other people's triumphs in order to reach your own goals. Believe in your natural and supernatural skills, and don't let doubt sneak into your spiritual life or activities.

3. <u>Think about the nature of consciousness.</u>

You are free to meditate as you walk through the park! You should not be limited to sitting or sleeping alone at home. This is a terrific method to suck up some natural energy while relaxing your mind and simply walking about the neighborhood. Because your mind is focused on physical activities, it will be able to free itself of stray notions that could deplete your vitality. When done correctly, meditation helps you to focus completely on raising your consciousness.

4. <u>Experiment with detecting the vibrancy of various products.</u>

This procedure is referred to as psychometry. All it takes is touching something to read its energy or contacting an object till you start to feel feelings coming from it. This is an excellent approach to learn about psychic talents and how to cultivate them.

What approach do you employ when performing psychometry?

- Before grabbing the stones, let your energy flow by rubbing your hands together.
- Breathe deeply and allow your energy to flow freely while holding the stone or stones in your palm. Don't be worried if you get tingling feelings in your hands.

Despite its absurd appearance, psychometry is a terrific activity for brain growth.

5. <u>Develop coping and overcoming strategies for your concerns.</u>

After deciding to discharge your psychic energy, you should be able to accept the consequences of your actions. While psychic and supernatural energy can be frightening, fear can make them difficult to detect. You should not be concerned if you predict something unexpected. Find a means to reconcile your disagreements with others around you.

To establish a psychological connection, you must be at ease with yourself and your surroundings. This can be accomplished by discussing any difficulties with others and attempting to avoid disputes totally. If a conflict arises, strive to address it constructively and explore how to do it kindly. Concentration is difficult when you are upset because anger depletes your spiritual force. As a result, if you wish to improve your psychic talents, you must first rid your environment of bad energy.

6. Maintain a positive frame of reference at all times.

Choose an activity that will provide you joy and happiness. Find something you enjoy doing that makes you happy, whatever it is! It is more difficult to create mental connections when you are scared because you lack concentration. As a result, let your concerns permeate deeper into your subconscious.

7. Make contact with your guiding spirit.

A spirit guide's job is to assist you in your spiritual growth and journey through life. It has been hand-picked for you and is now available on the internet. When you initially begin, it may be difficult to establish contact with your guiding mind, and you may need to spend some time meditating. After the first conversation, it's much easy to contact them.

8. Take care of your objectives.

We must pay attention to our dreams in order to speak with our inner voices and abilities. After your psychic skills have begun to develop and mature, it's possible that you'll begin manifesting yourself through dreams. Dreams can only be beneficial if we remember our past, our aspirations, and our development. You could keep a dream journal to measure your spiritual improvement.

9. Put your abilities to good use.

You'll need to practice every day to improve your talents because you're conditioning your mind to perform new behaviors. Regular practice will help you build new talents and push your thinking to the next level of sophistication. Practice in a calm, tranquil environment where you can concentrate successfully.

Is it important to have psychic powers in today's world?

Yes! This is due to your increased sensitivity to the opinions and feelings of others. While it takes time to develop psychic powers, the rewards of dedication are immense.

Chapter 31:
Becoming a Fun Empath

To be an empathic extrovert, all you need is love in your life. Contrary to popular belief, gregarious social butterfly types with an icy cold exterior aren't usually associated with extroverted empathy (and they're not always delighted to see you!).

Consider the following definition of empathy: the ability to understand and respond to another's feelings. The purpose of extroversion is to develop an extroverted or happy attitude toward life. Aha! "Attitude" is the crucial word in your statement. Attitude. Extroverted empathy refers to those who make a purposeful decision to spend time outside and feel positively (empathically) about others in order to assist the environment. These people have a tendency to put themselves in the shoes of others while showing no empathy for their own circumstances or situation. They understand how it feels to be in a situation where they cannot pass judgment or voice their feelings on either side of the debate.

Their desire to be extroverted empaths is so great that they falsely believe they can make friends with anyone, which could be detrimental to their circumstances. You must learn to reconcile your empathy with sound logic and express yourself when necessary, especially when the situation is critical. The trick is to utilize their emotional intelligence rather than allowing it to overwhelm them.

Extroverted Empathy Is A Subset Of Empathy.

Everything comes effortlessly to persons wired in this way: attentive listening, quick interpretation of social information, awareness of how things work, and contact with people from other backgrounds are all possible. You know how things affect you and can adapt to your emotional needs, allowing you to communicate with people efficiently. They have a strong intuition and can add to a conversation without even realizing it.

Even though extroverted empathy is less social than introverted empathy, they communicate fully via their thoughts rather than words. You'll only come across these folks by coincidence, and only if their minds haven't been impacted by other people's (often unfavorable) notions.

In a nutshell, these individuals are born with the ability and desire to comprehend others and their surroundings. They are content because they believe in the concepts of reciprocity and community engagement.

They are sensitive to other people's emotions but are unable to comprehend what or why they are feeling them. As a result, extroverted empathy requires a direct and visible evaluation of everything that happens in the surroundings. There is no reason to interact with another person unless absolutely necessary.

Learn something new about the future: Extroverted empathy cannot disregard their intuition or exterior evidence, even if they don't understand what they're witnessing. They immediately notice people as if they were forest dwellers. Observing someone's stride, facial expressions, and body language, as well as receiving an atmosphere from them that depicts the type of person they are on the inside, can help you determine if they are extroverted. Simply by looking at someone or a group of individuals, you may guess what will happen next.

People with this skill are extremely present in the moment and sensitive. Allowing others to walk in your shoes without passing judgment or taking your ideas personally enables them to solve difficulties more quickly than others. Others feel at ease and safe in a wide range of situations, from their deepest anxieties to those that enrage or dissatisfy them.

These folks are skilled at sensing and communicating the emotions of others. They routinely gather the information that others are unable to due to their empathy training. This information has helped them become exceptional communicators and translators, which has resulted in promotions, enhanced learning, a greater comprehension of the world, and personal development. Someone with this ability can help you calm down during a quarrel or empathize with you in stressful situations. They are popular because they allow for objective hearing.

Empathy's Undisclosed, Sulking Side

Being an extroverted empath has both advantages and disadvantages. To begin with, it is difficult for others to comprehend how bright and sensitive these people are when they are emotionless. Extruded empaths cling to their most private beliefs since they have been harmed repeatedly, and no one wants to approach them again. They may be aware of your behaviors, but they are unlikely to alert you of them. When people are frequently hurt, they cease connecting with others and bury their emotions. Extroverted empaths, on the other hand, approach life with the intention of fully appreciating it rather than trying to comprehend it.

These people attempt to establish a psychological barrier between themselves and others by suppressing their sentiments. They avoid connecting with others since they are unsure what to do. Bulimia or anorexia can occur when a person fully stops eating. You can spout one-line remark after one-line statement with no contribution to the conversation. They aren't going to express their emotions; thus, their silence says a lot. This is common in people who are exceptionally aware and sensitive but have bad childhood memories.

When extroverted empathies' moods improve, they devolve into addictions rather than expressing themselves to figure out why they're hurting in the first place. These individuals have a proclivity for concealing their genuine feelings beneath purportedly intriguing and superficial acts. People's emotions may be channeled via a big fountain of superficiality, and they would never learn to speak genuinely about their experiences.

Explaining the interior side of empathy is even more difficult than discussing the external aspect of empathy. Because their emotions are difficult to communicate, being an introverted empath may be both entertaining and unpleasant. If you're an introvert, you think about your feelings before expressing them to others. As a result, you will be able to perceive their inner emotions through their faces but not hear them.

Normally, an introverted empath appears ecstatic until you hit the wrong button and turn it off. They may be tremendously emotional one minute and appear fine the next, but only if they are not pushed over their breaking point. An introverted empath may appear cold, nonchalant, or even disdainful to individuals who do not grasp these concepts, and they may be true. This connects to the preceding example of trying to stop feelings at unsuitable times.

An introverted empath who learns to be outgoing will remain sensitive to the energy of others while attempting to ignore it. Because of their lack of empathy and sympathy, they may appear distant or carefree to those around them. They may also appear uneasy or hostile, but this is only because they are unaware of other people's feelings and are forced to push them away and ignore them until they learn how to behave appropriately.

Individuals who have witnessed or suffered sexual abuse, particularly older children and adults, may exhibit personality changes, notably in terms of emotional control and fearfulness while interacting with others.

If an abuser seduces or makes unwelcome overtures toward the victim, the victim may believe they are "pushing" the abuser to exploit them. Similarly, even if they did not initiate the split or commit any wrongdoing, they may feel responsible.

The Solutions: To whom should people with a higher EMPATH be referred for assistance?

While dealing with others can be challenging for an extroverted empath, there are strategies to help you relax and connect with them. The following are some strategies for assisting people in empathically communicating their sentiments to others:

Recognize when it is appropriate to express one's emotions (and when not to). Don't say anything if you're not sure how they'll react. Even if you are buddies with them, it is appealing to debate the matter with them. You, on the other hand, are uninterested in furthering the investigation. Have you experienced an especially tumultuous day? Have you experienced an especially tumultuous day? That's just great with me. You may always claim to be suffering from the blues later on (or something similar). If they inquire about your emotions, be open and honest, but don't expect them to comprehend immediately away. If you are asked again, attempt to provide a more detailed explanation to better understand.

Don't be hesitant to voice your strong feelings or opinions about something: Most extroverts are unafraid of expressing their thoughts and opinions in public. Be fearless and honest in your activities. When you have strong feelings about something, never be hesitant to express them clearly and totally. It would be excellent if you could avoid using offensive or judgemental language with other people at all times. This is the quickest method for silencing all emotions and communication.

Provide positive comments and encouragement: Even if you're not sure how someone will react, it's never a bad idea to provide positive feedback and encouragement. Simply reminding them of their efforts, even if they aren't always enough for others, or telling them they look great today, even if they're having a poor day, can be enough encouragement (unexpectedly). Giving positive feedback, for example, can have a big influence. If they're having a difficult day, all you have to do is smile and remind them of their worth. That is all that is required to provide them with the energy they require to get through the rest of the day without a doubt.

When an introvert is speaking, avoid interrupting or changing the subject; instead, listen more than you speak. Even though they appear to be rambling, it is critical to listen carefully and gently when an extrovert is speaking. Because most extroverts find silence unsettling, pay close attention to what they say when they do!

There is no need to pass judgment because the concept of extroverted empathy is not understood by everyone on the earth. They are not insane, and their experiences are true. Be patient and avoid casting judgment on them because you assume you are more knowledgeable than they are. Don't give up on an introvert just because something doesn't work right away. Teaching someone to accept others who are drastically different from themselves usually takes a long time and a lot of patience.

Discuss issues of common interest with them. When you're having a bad day or can't figure out what's wrong with your body, talk about something that interests you. Share your favorite piece of music with the group if it makes you feel better. If you find a movie or book that helps you relax, consider sharing it with others who might enjoy it as well. Extroverted empathizers will benefit from a quick discussion on the subject.

Conclusion

Empathy (also known as sympathy) is acknowledged as a psychic phenomenon related to clairvoyance due to the ability to accurately imagine another's spiritual experiences.

Empathy is defined as "knowing the depths of a sad or disappointed person's sentiments," "belonging to a trusted or unfairly insulted individual," or "a winner who appears to have the same feelings as others after performing his or her obligation."

No experience appears to be more fundamental than one received via life experiences because it demonstrates that our experiences are so close, if not identical, that recalling our own experiences in specific situations suffices to help grasp how the other person felt. Empathy-motivated activities, on the other hand, are far too rare.

We have all had hundreds of 'minor' incidents in which we have been injured or offended by inappropriate remarks, mockery, arrogance, or contempt... In each situation, the reason is the same: egoism (the belief that I am the only person who is significant and deserving of, say, compassion) or, at the very least, egotism (the conviction that I am the only one who is deserving of, say, compassion) (i.e., consider myself the "center of the world" that others have to comply with).

Your social skills influence how you interact with your family, friends, coworkers, and love partners.

It is normal to feel awful about a situation and respond by aiding others in any way we can. Empathy does not always work; it has the potential to fail. It is necessary for a person's social existence.

In layman's terms, it comprises "placing yourself in the shoes of another," "feeling and absorbing what you and the rest of the world experience from their perspective," and "putting yourself in the shoes of another." You'll never understand why someone behaved or acted the way they did until you put yourself in their shoes and see things through their eyes.

According to the definition, empathy is "psychological identification with or vicarious experience of another person's feelings, thoughts, or attitudes. Sympathy is the expression of grief for another person's suffering to convey solace, sympathy, or sadness.